# THE TRUTH BEHIND EPSTEIN-BARR VIRUS

The Truth Behind Epstein-Barr Virus

*The Multi-Dimensional Virus Creating Mental, Physical & Spiritual Dysfunction*

Tracey Gillies

©2024 All Rights Reserved. No portion of this book may be reproduced, stored in a retrieval system, or transmitted in any form or by any means—electronic, mechanical, photocopy, recording, scanning, or other—except for brief quotations in critical reviews or articles without the prior permission of the author.

Published by Game Changer Publishing

Paperback ISBN: 978-1-965653-02-9
Hardcover ISBN: 978-1-965653-03-6
Digital ISBN: 978-1-965653-04-3

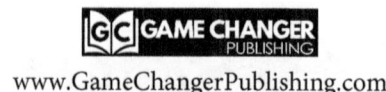

www.GameChangerPublishing.com

# DEDICATION

I dedicate this book to my family: Greg, Georgie, Charlee, Jones, Lola, and Hunter. Without your love and support, this journey would not have been possible.

To my husband Greg:
Thank you for loving me through it all. My elevation would not have been possible without yours, so I thank you for coming on this journey with me. Thank you for always supporting me, for keeping my mind sound by allowing me to share every single step of my journey—into the darkest places and back—with you, and for believing in me when I felt I might falter. Thank you for being my biggest fan.

# Read This First

Just to say thanks for buying and reading my book, I would like to gift you more resources, no strings attached!

**ACCESS TO MY FREE COMMUNITY + MINI-COURSE**

To help you gain more knowledge on *The Truth Behind Epstein-Barr Virus* plus access to additional learnings, resources, and a community to support your healing and transformation journey! Please scan the QR code for the above gifts!

**Scan the QR Code:**

# The Truth Behind Epstein-Barr Virus

*The Multi-Dimensional Virus Creating Mental, Physical & Spiritual Dysfunction*

**Tracey Gillies**

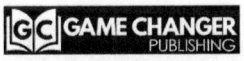

www.GameChangerPublishing.com

# Foreword

No one has had the exposure to Tracey's crazy journey like I have!

I'm Greg, Tracey's husband. I'm proud to be writing the foreword of her first book, and I'm equally proud of Tracey's resilience and dedication to herself in becoming the wife, mother, healer, and coach that she is.

Although this very important book is on *The Truth Behind Epstein-Barr Virus* and the learnings, gifts and healing abilities Tracey has developed around EBV, it is only one area of her extraordinary abilities.

As you read this book, I'm sure you'll have many "aha" moments, "wow" moments, not only about EBV, but about all aspects of healing, transformation, and gaining a deeper understanding of your own truths as a multidimensional being.

I've been exposed to so many events, experiences and personal changes through Tracey that have completely changed who I am and the paradigm of what I know and believe to be the truth of life.

Throughout Tracey's journey of healing and unlocking her highest gifts, we experienced some very dark times. Many times, I worried and thought I was going to lose her as she got really sick and was exposed to some dark energy and entities I would never wish upon anyone.

As you will learn in this book and from Tracey's stories, her profound healing gifts are due to her ability to command the highest dark energy and dark entities.

This book is extremely important as most of the world's population is living with some level of mental, physical, and spiritual dysfunction, resulting in unprecedented levels of mysterious illness, disease, ill health, and disconnection... you will learn that EBV is the deepest underlying cause of 95% of it all.

The world needs to evolve, and more and more people like Tracey need to unlock their highest gifts to help the world evolve. I hope you gain all the answers you are searching for and that the information in this book helps you on a journey of healing and living your best life.

As each person heals and evolves, so do we all!

– Greg Gillies

# Table of Contents

Introduction ..................................................................................... 1

Chapter 1 – Understanding EBV and Its Pathway to Creating So Much Destruction .................................................. 5

Chapter 2 – My Story: Healing From EBV ............................... 15

Chapter 3 – Mind: How EBV Affects the Brain ........................ 41

Chapter 4 – Body: How EBV Affects the Body ........................ 57

Chapter 5 – Spirit: Vibrational Frequencies and Energy .......... 77

Chapter 6 – Entities ................................................................ 105

Chapter 7 – Transformation Is the Key to Healing EBV for Good ... 139

Chapter 8 – EBV Is a Collective Disease ................................. 157

Conclusion ............................................................................... 171

A Special Thank You .............................................................. 175

# Introduction

Epstein-Barr virus (EBV) is a silent epidemic, a virus that creates significant destruction in its wake. Unfortunately, in my experience, by the time a person starts to link EBV to their health decline, it has often progressed to a point where it is very difficult to unwind. The body is very good at compensating for itself, masking issues, and redirecting resources repeatedly until there are no more resources to extend.

What you need to understand is that Epstein-Barr virus is a multidimensional virus with many layers, as well as energetic associations. It creates so much dysfunction and disconnection across all levels of a person's being: mind, body, and soul.

I have seen people chase the virus for decades, trying one approach, one healing protocol after another, without success. Everything has a purpose and a reason for existing; EBV and its heightened levels in each person's body are no different.

When it comes to healing, you have to find the true underlying cause and heal from that, or all else is simply a "Band-Aid" fix. Until you understand the truth behind EBV's existence specifically for you, you will be in an endless loop. Maybe you will get a reprieve and have the virus reduce, but it will simply wait for another stressful point in your life to occur and recreate itself over and over again, as this is what the virus is programmed to do.

As you read through this book, you will learn how EBV affects a person multi-dimensionally. The book is structured to take you through all the different dimensions and information. You will learn:

- How the second dimension, the realm of viruses, is shifting due to collective instability.
- The pathway to decline in a person's physical body and the interlinks that are important when it comes to trying to heal physically from the virus.
- How the brain plays the most critical role in healing the past.
- How our stress responses and life's traumas play an intricate role in feeding the virus.
- How to achieve lasting healing, neurological rebalancing, and repair as a gateway to expanded consciousness, facilitating deep healing within the body's organs and glands.
- Why certain protocols you have tried for healing are not creating lasting change.
- How EBV is symbolic of a world on the brink of disorder and interlinked with human expansion, transformation, and ultimately soul reconnection.
- How EBV is interlinked with dark energies and dark entities.
- To heal Epstein-Barr virus, you have to learn how to restore balance within, breaking all energetic ties in your life and your past to the virus.

Who am I to make such claims?

My name is Tracey Gillies, and I am an energy and spiritual healer who specialises in two things: Epstein-Barr virus and dark energy and dark entity interference (demonic and multi-dimensional).

I will tell you about my pathway to healing myself from EBV. Through this pathway, I unlocked the most extraordinary and powerful spiritual gifts, ones that now allow me to heal others from these very things.

Once upon a time, when I was not as wise, I would have told you all the blame lies with the virus. This would be the easiest thing to think. We live in a world that loves to create one face to a dark presence, to abdicate responsibility, a world of quick fixes and instant gratification. Through healing myself from EBV, I learned the story was never simply that of a virus.

My knowledge does not come from books; it comes from healing myself, reverse engineering the virus, and always working at the deepest levels of a person's mind, body, and soul to create lasting and true transformation.

I hope this book offers many things: hope and faith, answers and awareness. But more so, I hope it acts as a catalyst for activation in your energetic field, awakening memories of path progression and the next steps in healing.

In the past, I have read many books that have acted as pivotal points in my healing journey, offering more than awareness. These books created subtle shifts in my energetic field, which often felt like a tingling sensation, a confirmation that the information was resonating at a deeper level within me.

New awareness is key to creating healing and change.

CHAPTER 1

# Understanding EBV and Its Pathway to Creating So Much Destruction

I didn't realise that a virus that had been hosted in my body for decades could create so many restrictions for me later in life. However, now that I understand how this virus works, I'm wiser to know that my life, my fears, and my stress played a role in compounding it.

Epstein-Barr virus has actually been around for a very, very long time. At one point, it was in balance, just as the world around us was. There are many contributing factors related to how we're living and our internal stress responses that have caused EBV to morph into something that causes so much destruction at all levels of mind, body, and soul.

But first, in order to really understand EBV, you have to comprehend what it is and how it works.

Epstein-Barr virus is part of the herpes virus family, and it's one of the most common human viruses. It's human herpesvirus 4, and 95% of the world's population has it. It causes an infection called glandular fever, also known as mononucleosis (mono).

So, how do people contract Epstein-Barr virus? It's passed through bodily fluids and saliva. This is why glandular fever, or mono, has been nicknamed "the kissing disease." A lot of people contract it in their teenage years, but it's also passed in utero to unborn babies.

So how would you know if you have it? Some people can be asymptomatic. I know with my children, I passed EBV to them in utero, and they didn't show any symptoms until years later. Until the virus gets activated, many people don't even realise they've had it. Some people know they've had glandular fever, perhaps severely, during their teenage years. Otherwise, it could present as swollen glands, headaches, fever, or simply feel like a common flu, and many people don't realise they've had it. They also may not realise that it's the underlying cause of their health concerns even decades later.

Are there tests for EBV? Yes, you can request a blood test from your doctor. The results will indicate whether your body has antibodies to EBV, showing that you've had it at some point. However, the results might also indicate that you either no longer have it or that it's inactive, which is where the real problem lies. This can be confusing for people, as they may think it can't be causing their current health concerns.

Conditions like fatigue, adrenal issues, thyroid issues, brain fog, digestive issues, hormonal imbalance, inflammation, mystery illnesses, and even restrictions in spiritual connection can all be late-stage manifestations of a body and mind that have become dysfunctional due to an ever-growing virus.

The confusing thing about test results is that they often show a heightened level of EBV. You may be told you are in a reactivation state, but even after the reactivation clears, it does not mean Epstein-Barr virus has declined in your body. Many people think they are in remission, but it does not work like that. By the time you are experiencing reactivation, you will be in the much later stages of EBV, where the virus will be compromising nearly every single organ and gland in your body as well as inflaming your central nervous system, causing further health decline.

Reactivations are like a tipping point. Seemingly minor changes in life circumstances, another illness, or extra stress on the immune system or central nervous system, which the body can no longer handle due to the high viral load, can lead to the virus returning to the active infection stage.

I'm going to show you how Epstein-Barr virus actually affects the body in different stages and help you understand that it is classified as an opportunistic virus. This is the danger with it. Essentially, you've had it at some point, and your body has initiated an immune response, making it seem like you don't really have it anymore. But EBV never leaves a person's body.

In Stage 1, it will sit in the liver and spleen because it feeds off toxicity. It loves mercury, dioxins, and many other toxins, and it lays in wait. It's like it's hiding, and it waits until you are dealing with some other immune stress or response. Women tend to suffer from it more, or maybe they are more aware of their suffering because they have so much going on physically that their bodies have to deal with, like monthly cycles, pregnancy, having a baby, and sleep deprivation. But it actually affects the liver detoxification pathway, specifically methylation, which is the pathway for processing hormones.

When I was struggling to understand what was going on with my health and searching for answers, I was told it was depression. However, I felt it was more hormonal because it aligned with my monthly cycle. One therapist once told me I was a poor methylator, which means I didn't process hormones properly, and I was given a supplement to try and alleviate the symptoms.

But what's really going on, and the underlying cause, is that Epstein-Barr virus is actually preventing that liver detoxification pathway from functioning correctly. I think that's why women tend to notice the symptoms more, but it does affect men just as much. I have worked with hundreds of men, and 95% of them had high levels of EBV due to their stress levels.

So, when it reaches Stage 2, remembering it lies and waits for life to happen—maybe a marriage breakup, a death, or other stressful events. It then attacks the thyroid. In fact, 95% of thyroid dysfunction is caused by Epstein-Barr virus.

Many people are told by doctors that their body is attacking itself, that it's an autoimmune response attacking the thyroid. But that's not what's actually happening. The immune system is attacking EBV at a cellular level.

It is trying to eradicate a virus that has burrowed in and is compromising the thyroid's function. Many people don't understand how important the thyroid is. It monitors long-wave frequencies in the body and oversees the functioning of many other organs and glands.

Once the thyroid is compromised, Epstein-Barr virus can compromise pretty much every single organ and gland in the body. Many people come to me with adrenal issues, thyroid problems, or endocrine system dysfunctions responsible for hormone function. But it's actually EBV causing these issues, and they are just symptomatic of it.

In working with people, I have found that it can affect every single structure in the body except the small intestine or bladder. It can cause destruction in nearly every gland, organ, and structure in the mind and body. It compromises key structures critical for healing and supporting the body, including the liver and its detoxification pathways, as well as creating huge stress on a person's lymphatic system.

The next stage, Stage 3, is really serious. This is when Epstein-Barr virus crosses the blood-brain barrier. It can do this by attaching to mercury and using it as a transport mechanism. Once EBV crosses the blood-brain barrier, it attacks and inflames the central nervous system, affecting neurotransmitters, neurological structures, and many other brain functions that support the neurons, the perineural system, and the cranial respiratory system.

Unfortunately, mercury is a neurotoxin that can confuse the brain into thinking it doesn't have enough mercury. So, your body will continually try to retain more and more mercury, creating higher mercury levels and enabling Epstein-Barr virus to continue to build. It's not as simple as detox or heavy metal supplementation because if your brain is in conflict and thinks it needs mercury, you have to heal the neurological confusion first.

The brain is the top organisational structure in our body and plays a significant role in healing from EBV. This is why I have dedicated an entire chapter to this topic.

As Epstein-Barr virus builds, it wreaks havoc on the central nervous system. It can affect a number of different nerves and nerve endings.

You have various nerves, such as the vagus nerve, which plays a big role in the central nervous system, but there are also nerves in your face. People might complain of tingling or even burning sensations in their faces. Another nerve runs down your lungs and heart, which might cause symptoms like heart palpitations, heart issues, breathing problems, or even panic attacks. This compounds stress and Sympathetic Nervous System Dominance (SNSD), making it a breeding ground for all illnesses and diseases.

That's right, Epstein-Barr virus has been linked to many neurological illnesses, declines, and diseases, including Alzheimer's, Parkinson's, and cancer.

Now that you understand how Epstein-Barr virus affects the brain and its neurological structures, I'd like to touch on how it then affects the body's autonomic nervous system. The brain, as the top organisational structure of the human body, also controls the autonomic nervous system, which is responsible for all the automatic processes that happen in our body, like breathing, heartbeat, digestion, and blood pressure.

There are two sides to the autonomic nervous system:

1. **Sympathetic Nervous System:** When we are in this state, our body pushes blood flow away from our major organs and into our muscles as we gear up for activity. This is a key function for humans. However, when the sympathetic nervous system is overactive, it can lead to Sympathetic Nervous System Dominance.
2. **Parasympathetic Nervous System:** This is the state we activate when we are resting and relaxed. In this state, blood flows back to the organs and glands, enabling our systems to heal and repair.

When we are in balance, we should be able to transition between these two states for optimal health and well-being. Unfortunately, due to many factors, including Epstein-Barr virus and compounded deep survival stress, we lose the ability to transition between these two states. This leaves 95% of the world's population living in a state known as Sympathetic Nervous System Dominance.

This is where the real problem begins. Because Epstein-Barr virus compromises, inflames, and attacks the entire central nervous system, it pushes us deeper into a state called Sympathetic Nervous System Dominance, which then affects our endocrine system, the hormonal response system of our body. What it does is signal our adrenal glands to produce cortisol. Cortisol is the body's response to stress or danger, and it is a necessary response. However, when we are stuck in this deep state of stress and are overproducing cortisol, it causes significant damage to the body.

I see many people who come to me, and despite eating well and doing all the right things, their bodies are not responding. The reason for this is that when we overproduce cortisol, it changes our entire metabolism to suit a survival stress state. We crave fast-burning foods like sugars, refined carbs, alcohol, and caffeine. It's not just because we want these things; it's because, in this state, our body needs them to function. We are literally stuck in fight-or-flight mode, and our body thinks it needs fast-burning food to survive. Even when we eat well, like proteins and fats, our body cannot digest these foods properly, leading to fermentation and increased inflammation. This is actually the pathway to all diseases.

Many people say that heart disease or other illnesses run in their family. While there may be a genetic predisposition to certain illnesses or diseases, the pathway to get there is the same. When we hold so much stress neurologically, we get stuck in Sympathetic Nervous System

Dominance, losing our ability to heal and repair, and we slowly decline. Again, it is Epstein-Barr virus pushing us deeper into stress and holding us there.

You can't heal from Epstein-Barr virus until you heal from deep survival stress first. EBV, being an opportunistic virus, uses our own body against us. It uses our own stress responses against us. It lies in wait for stress to happen, causing a compounding effect in the body. When your body is busy dealing with another threat—whether a physical threat, an illness, the flu, or a heightened stress event in life (such as a marriage breakdown, a death, losing a job, or high bills)—the virus takes advantage. We live in a busy world with many demands, and there are many things that cause us stress. It's almost like the world has changed, but our brain has not. To understand how the brain functions and what it links stress to, you need to understand brain development. We will cover this in Chapter 3, which focuses on how the Epstein-Barr virus affects our mind and brain function. But first, let me tell you about my journey with EBV.

## Chapter Summary

In this chapter, I have provided an overview of Epstein-Barr virus and how it creates significant damage and dysfunction across a person's mind, body, and soul. I explained that EBV is a multi-dimensional virus that affects a person on all levels of their being. The chapter outlines what the reader will learn throughout the book, including how stress responses and traumas feed the virus, the importance of neurological rebalancing, and the connection between EBV, dark energies and entities, and human transformation. I also introduce myself and my expertise in healing EBV and dark energy/entity interference.

## CHAPTER 2

# My Story: Healing From EBV

I actually have two stories to share with you throughout this book, but I'd like to start by sharing my story of serious health decline and my journey to learning about and healing from Epstein-Barr virus.

I felt like my health decline really started after having my first child in 2008. Becoming a mother is a life-changing event in so many ways, from being responsible for another life to feeling completely out of your depth, dealing with stress, sleep deprivation, second-guessing everything, and learning how to take care of a little baby. We lived far away from our entire family and did not have any support, which compounded the demands and pressure, leaving no end in sight and no one to step in and save me or offer me a much-needed break.

I loved being a mom, but I don't think I realised at the time how my health had already been in decline for many years, and having a baby compounded this. Georgie had colic, although it took me a while to understand this. Essentially, colic is a label that simply means your baby cries and is unsettled a lot, usually passed off as a digestive disturbance.

"Crying and unsettled" was an understatement. She would scream for five to six hours a night, and I tried everything to settle her. I didn't know what to do. Every time I put her down to sleep, she would wake up again within minutes, until around 1–2 a.m., when she would sleep soundly until about 5 a.m. This was our nightly routine.

I dreaded the witching hour from around 6 p.m. until 1 a.m. It was a nightmare. I was exhausted, mentally and physically, and without any family support, it was just me and my husband fumbling through life. Looking back, it was definitely digestive discomfort, as I had passed my foundation for health to her, meaning she inherited my microbiome, my ill health, and my digestive issues. Knowing what I know now about health and healing, I wish I had had a healthier platform for having children and imparting knowledge and wisdom, as well as a blueprint for health, to them.

But this was not the case. My health declined rapidly. I was exhausted mentally and physically but had no choice but to keep going. That first year was the hardest for me. I remember going to the doctor near the end of the first year, just before Georgie turned one. I felt like something wasn't right with me. I was struggling on so many levels, dealing with fatigue, mood swings, hormonal imbalance, and mental strain. I felt as though something was wrong with me beyond simply being a new mom struggling with life.

I think I went back numerous times, and each time, they simply said it was postnatal depression. I was told I was clinically depressed and to take medication.

I've always loved natural therapies and have tried many different things, so for me, taking medication wasn't the answer. I felt that when life is really hard, you can't just take a pill to make it better. That was just how I felt.

So, I really had to push them to do more tests and to listen to my concerns. Once the blood tests came back, they showed that I had Epstein-Barr virus and had experienced a reactivation of it, resulting in glandular fever for around three to four months. The tests also showed that I had contracted a very severe food poisoning called toxoplasmosis, which can last around three months and make someone feel physically ill.

I felt happy that there was a real physical reason for how I had been feeling, that it was not all in my head. So, for me, that was enough to think, *Well, no wonder I'm feeling really down. I've got a baby with colic, I've got so much stress, and I'm exhausted.* There were physical reasons, and I just kind of soldiered on as I always had before.

Then, after my second child was born, she had digestive issues, too. Later on, I realised she was lactose intolerant. She would scream in pain at night, and in the end, to try and alleviate stress as well as get some sleep, I co-slept with her. This helped a little, but again, I was surviving on nothing, next to no sleep, and now I had not one but two children—a demanding toddler and a newborn baby.

I started to see more issues in my health. Not just being exhausted; at this point, I think I had simply gotten used to this being my new normal.

I had a lot of digestive issues. To combat my baby's lactose intolerance, I cut out all dairy from my diet. Anyone would think this change would have created healing in my body and started to restore my health, but it only seemed to compound it. In the end, it resulted in me getting thrush—endless thrush, over and over. It was unbearable. I think the change in my diet created an imbalance elsewhere. I was desperate to heal myself, not just for my sake but for my baby's as well. I was constantly trying endless health diets, adding things to my diet, and taking things out.

I know this place better than anyone with good health. I felt like I was endlessly fumbling in the dark. You name it, I have tried it. I was dedicated to whatever cause might be the thing to help.

Once again, I turned to natural therapies, supplementation, and diet—whatever it took, I was willing to do it.

Then, the icing on the cake, or should I say the nail in the coffin, was when I had my third child. Before this, I was somehow keeping my head just above water.

Jones, my third child, was my easiest, probably because I had made many changes in my health and diet. I knew what to do with a baby, and I knew what to cut out of my diet through breastfeeding, which made a huge difference, as I had learned this with my other two.

Although motherhood is never easy, adding more to the mix—more demands, more sleep deprivation—I was very proud of myself. I had breastfed all my children; in fact, I had still been breastfeeding Charlee right up to being eight months pregnant with Jones.

When Jones was around three months old, I really hit a breaking point. I couldn't function by pushing through as I had been. I remember starting to have what felt like panic attacks. I would be out with my three children, and the overwhelm became too much, especially if I was in a noisy, stressful environment.

Looking back now and considering what I know about EBV, mental health, and the physical body, I can see that all my pieces were missing. I was simply waiting to break. Adrenals taken to the brink of exhaustion over and over eventually create a final phase, which is like a collapse—adrenal burnout. Here I was in this place; it was so dark, and I didn't even know how to pull myself out of it.

This is the place of a mental breakdown. I have been to these places in myself, and I would never wish this upon anyone.

I went back to the doctor. Leading up to this, the only conversations they would entertain were that I was depressed and needed to go on medication. In fact, after each child in the hospital, I was put on a watch list as I was high risk due to feeling this way after my first was born.

It was a really, really scary time in my life. I remember crying to my mum on the phone, saying I didn't want to be here anymore, and she was pleading with me to take medication. My husband was also swaying to this side, as he could see I was not coping with life. It felt unmanageable.

Once again, I just knew in my heart of hearts that this was not the answer.

At this point, I made a very vulnerable post on social media asking for advice and help. I knew I wasn't depressed because my mood swings, feelings of being completely overwhelmed, extreme mood shifts, and depletion aligned with my monthly cycle. I could be struggling one week and then back to my normally bubbly self the next, where my life was manageable. This did not feel like depression to me; it felt more like a hormonal imbalance.

I received a lot of beautiful responses, and the ones I appreciated the most were from other women struggling with the exact same issues. It let me know I was not alone. Many recommendations specifically focused on balancing hormones, and one of them was Traditional Chinese Medicine (TCM).

So, I sought out a traditional Chinese herbalist. He took a holistic look at my life and said he had never seen anyone with more stress than me. I had three kids under the age of five, my husband travelled overseas for work all the time, and we had no family support, as they all lived back in New Zealand. It meant there was no break, no end in sight, and my health and stress had compounded over the past four and a half years. All my symptoms were a result of adrenal exhaustion/burnout. This was the answer at the time, and while it was correct, I have learned that you can't simply focus on one area of the body or health to restore it. Adrenal burnout was part of a much bigger picture.

The herbalist gave me some herbs to support my adrenals, and being seen and validated made me feel much better. There was a reason for my symptoms, and if I could find the reasons, I could ultimately find the solution.

I started taking a tonic, and it helped slightly. I will admit that once I started trying to recover my adrenals, I got sick constantly. I was reassured it was all part of the healing process, so once more, I kept moving forward, or at least trying to.

I was prepared to do whatever it took to help myself heal, although simply taking a tonic felt like a very long road ahead, especially when I was dealing with so much daily business and stress.

Then, I felt like I got the break of my life—something that I thought was going to fix everything and drastically change my life.

My husband got offered a contract to move to Singapore for his career, and we were all to go as a family.

Life in Singapore, as an expat wife, was a complete contrast to my life in Australia.

The lifestyle there includes having a live-in maid, referred to as a domestic helper. I wouldn't need to work; in fact, I wasn't allowed to work on the visa that we were on.

My life was about to change drastically. I always said if only I didn't have these boring, stressful mummy jobs anymore, I would be fine; life would be completely different for me. So, we moved to Singapore, had a live-in domestic helper, and lived in a resort-style condo that seemed like something out of a movie, like a holiday resort. There was an Olympic-sized swimming pool, a children's pool and sauna, six tennis courts, two squash courts, a gym, three playgrounds, BBQ areas, and it even had its own shop. It was amazing!

I thought I was going to be this amazing person with so much time on my hands, as my biggest excuse for being overrun was the lack of time. But I wasn't this amazing person. While I seemed less stressed, played with my children, went to the gym, relaxed, and had a social life, deep down, I still felt disconnected, unhappy, lonely, and sad within myself.

It was a strange place to be, getting everything I thought would bring happiness and health, yet feeling like there were still pieces missing. I also felt like I couldn't tell anyone this because, from the outside looking in, my life looked magical, with nothing to complain about. And yet, I felt really disconnected and like something was missing. It was really hard because I now had all the time in the world. I thought I was going to be this amazing person. I did do all these things to work on myself, yet I couldn't really tell people how miserable and unhappy I was because I looked like I had it all.

During this time, I wasn't that good to myself. I ate well and exercised but often turned to alcohol as a way to find joy and happiness. It had become a coping mechanism for me, although most of the people I surrounded myself with drank, so at that point in time, I did not really question my choices.

We were meant to stay in Singapore long term; my husband's contract was for ten years plus.

But two years later, the contract abruptly ended, and we found ourselves back in Australia. All the demands piled up again, and with them, the stress.

While I had been in Singapore, I knew I wasn't that happy, but due to the lifestyle, I thought I had resolved many of my issues. Once the stress compounded again, it didn't even take two months to realise just what a terrible place I was truly in.

It felt like déjà vu. How did I end up here again?

I thought I had worked on myself and that my time in Singapore had alleviated and resolved the past. How wrong I was.

I once again went back to what I did best: search for answers. At the time, my answer was to double down—I would just be better, eat better, work out harder, and add more to my to-do list. Organisation was the key, and of course, I would try more natural therapies and healing modalities.

When I was in Singapore, I saw dietitians, hypnotherapists, and an osteopath. I took meditation courses and had so much free time to myself.

Since I had seen an osteopath in Singapore who did kinesiology to test supplements, I thought this was what I would try next.

I found a kinesiologist, and when I called her, I asked if she would test some supplements for me and tell me what I could take to improve my health and reduce my stress.

She was lovely and said that while that wasn't really what she did, I should bring my supplements along, and she would test them along with a number of other things.

I went to see her. She was trained in a modality called Advanced Holistic Kinesiology and used other energy-healing techniques. She tested my supplements but also did an energetic audit of several of my organs and glands as part of my first healing session.

She said that if my lungs were not functioning at the level they were, she would have said my body was going into shutdown and was holding so much stress and misalignments.

It felt confronting to realise I was right back in the same place; I really hadn't healed anything. I remember crying to my husband and saying, "Oh my God, I thought I had fixed this, and I haven't. I really have to fix it once and for all. I have to heal my life."

I saw this therapist for around three months, which had a huge impact on me, both mentally and physically.

Then, in one session, she said that I needed to do something for myself. I had lost myself in being a mom, and although I loved my children, I felt as though I had sacrificed a lot to meet everyone else's needs.

When she said this to me, I instantly replied that I wanted to do what she was doing. I felt so blessed, as the course was in Brisbane, the city I lived in, and it was only 15 minutes from home.

I later found out that Australia and New Zealand are the most advanced in this therapy in the world, and the head trainer had created a lot of the course content himself. He was an exceptional man with exceptional talent.

It was like the stars all aligned for me to learn this amazing modality. It is one of the most advanced and in-depth courses in the world, and it felt like everything just fell into place for me.

I never thought I was going to heal people or be a healer. I just had a lot to heal in myself. It felt aligned, as I had always been interested in natural therapies for myself and others. In fact, on many occasions, I had roped my husband into attending various healing sessions, many of which we laugh about to this day.

Learning Advanced Holistic Kinesiology became a passion, and I fell in love with it!

The course was really involved and gave me an amazing foundation and understanding of the physical body, organs, and glands, how to work with them at a health level, neurological structures, and the interplay they have on a person's physical health and healing. The most powerful side of all is energy and our spiritual and soul connection. Learning about this opened my mind to a new and powerful world that I didn't even realise existed.

Until this point, I didn't even realise that we were spiritual beings having a human experience. I didn't realise the power of energy. I became obsessed.

Normally, with this particular healing therapy, you would lie on a table in front of a therapist who would use your muscles to get an indication, tapping into your central nervous system and something called your innate intelligence. This allows the therapist to see where you are holding stress, as the muscular feedback receives a response directly from the central nervous system. It's almost like a yes or no response, enabling you to learn how to read the body and its energetics. It also directly connects with a person's innate intelligence, this inherent knowing, body wisdom—call it what you like. It knows exactly what we need to be in optimal physical, mental, emotional, and spiritual alignment.

We all have this inherent knowing, and if we can simply hear this truth, it allows us to tap into the calling of our soul, and the possibilities are endless. Kinesiology is also like a framework; later on, I realised that whatever I learned could simply be added to this amazing, energetic database of skills and knowledge.

I was taught how to find areas that are holding stress, not just in a person's physical body in the form of dysfunction in organs, glands, body structures, and systems, but also stress held at the level of the mind, structures recycling the past, neurological frameworks in decline, as well as conflict held in the form of outdated belief systems, limited viewpoints, and obsolete versions of self. Then, we work at the level of the soul to harmonise past lifetime information and soul restrictions, and we use the reconnective power of the soul as a regulation of all energetic structures. By balancing the energetic information around this to release stress or misalignment throughout mind, body, and soul, we have the most amazing ability to self-heal and come back into balance within ourselves.

I loved it, and I just wanted to practise all the time. Plus, I had so many things to heal within myself, so learning and healing went hand in hand.

At this point, my children were still very young, and when I practised on them, they didn't want to lie still on a table. So, I started working through something called energetic surrogacy, which involves bringing their energy into my body and working through myself, using my own body as a tool to heal another. Anything that I changed or healed would reflect in their physical bodies.

The balance between healing my family and the endless healing work I needed to do on myself was crucial. Whenever I learned a new process or protocol, I would simply repeat it over and over in my own body, my own energetics, getting practice while also healing more and more. I would then repeat this process for each family member.

This enhanced my skills and learning and became my platform for healing. I started to work with all my clients in this way. As I developed more and more abilities, I could do more and more by working in this way, as it allowed me to bypass a person's conscious mind. Working in this way has not been easy and is a skill in itself to learn and master. It's taken me years and years to develop these skills. If you understand how energy works, you know that if anything resonated with me, it would heighten my restrictions and resonate with my issues, which meant I had to continually work on myself. At the end of every session, I would have to say there would be no negative side effects for me, though there were many over many years.

I have done more work on myself than people would do in lifetimes, clearing restrictions so I could use my body as a tool—a fine-tuned tool that could hold other people's issues and illnesses without compromising myself.

Working in this way was not without sacrifice. I spent many years being sick. My husband would often ask why I chose to work this way. For me, I loved it. If I was having a hard time or became sick through resonance, it simply meant I had more work to do and more restrictions to release.

So, I had that journey through learning and training in Advanced Holistic Kinesiology, healing myself at the time. But I also had another journey, realising I had very special gifts with dark energy and dark entities.

I've clinically trained in quite a few different modalities.

I've learned Holographic Kinetics, soul realignment, and many other modalities and techniques in energy healing.

When I first started studying kinesiology, the head trainer, who is one of the best in the world and has created his own advanced curriculum, remarked that it was strange how many dark energies and dark entities were attached to me.

He only knew a fraction of it, as I didn't realise at the time that I had gifts—"soul gifts"—that can't be taught. It took me a long time to get a handle on these gifts because I didn't have many people who could help me. It was as if there wasn't a roadmap for what I had to deal with. I had these amazing abilities with healing that I didn't recognise because dark energy and dark entities like to stifle that in a person.

It was a lengthy process for me to heal myself and reclaim these gifts. I go into more detail in the chapter on entities about my path and progression with this. I have so many stories to share on this topic; some are extreme and may sound a little unbelievable. One day, I will write another book dedicated to dark energy and dark entities.

This is why I spoke about having two different stories. The person I once was seemed to fade into the background, and a new form of myself emerged through healing and reclaiming my gifts. My knowledge about Epstein-Barr virus, as well as entity interference, does not come from formal learnings; it comes from my own life experiences, healing myself and reclaiming the highest pieces/aspects of my soul.

My journey has led me to work at higher and higher levels. All of this came through self-development as well as working with and healing people.

My journey felt extreme because when you learn any form of energetic work, your energetic systems want to test it. As I progressed in the course and expanded my learning, each new lesson led me to more healing, finding more and more things to heal. It was amazing how my energetics worked. There were many times that things replayed in my body so I could heal them in the correct way. My body recreated the miscarriage of a baby from when I was younger. It was as if I had to relive this experience to resolve it properly, harmonise the trauma, and turn pain into growth and transformation. My body did the same with EBV. I had a monumental flare-up, and it resurfaced once again. Up until this point, I had not realised that it was one of the greatest underlying issues in my health degeneration.

With my increasing skills and knowledge of the physical body and structures, as well as an in-depth understanding of the brain, I was able to track the virus and its stages. I also began reading more information about it, including resources like the Medical Medium. As my conscious awareness started to look deeper at this virus in my own body, I began to see amazing interconnections with the virus, the body, and the brain. I started understanding it in a deeper way, not just reciting information but seeing the consequences and the severity of its destruction in the body's organs and glands, neurological structures, and even its interplay with the spiritual realms.

I developed a structure and protocol for reducing the virus. At this point, I was starting to work with more and more clients and realised they all had Epstein-Barr virus, some more severe than others.

Although I was more focused on transformation and spiritual development, healing was certainly a key piece. To create a profound transformation for a client, I had to work simultaneously across all levels: mind, body, and soul. To create change and transformation, I always had to reduce and help them recover from Epstein-Barr virus to make expanded consciousness a possibility.

If EBV stayed in a person's body and mind, it presented the opportunity to derail a life, create huge health restrictions, and set a pathway to decline. This is when I realised that healing a person from Epstein-Barr virus was more about transformation, changing the trajectory of their life. There was a bigger picture than just physical decline involved.

Over time, I've had clients come to me for various reasons. One client had migraines her whole life. She didn't come to me for that; she came to transform her life. By default, it was actually Epstein-Barr virus that was the issue, specifically affecting her methylation pathway. Through healing EBV, she got rid of her migraines. Her therapist contacted me, expressing his astonishment at the outcome and was surprised to learn that EBV was the primary cause behind it.

I had another client who had parasites from the food they ate in Bali 20 years earlier. It had ruined their life because their whole digestive system was under so much stress, and they couldn't eat certain things, causing a lot of anxiety. They had seen specialist after specialist, but it was Epstein-Barr virus that I had to heal to restore their digestive system.

I've had clients with Lyme disease who had seen numerous specialists in the medical industry and couldn't get rid of it. But it was Epstein-Barr virus holding the Lyme disease in place.

Time and time again, I realised that to transform people's lives and heal all the symptoms they came to me for, I had to work with Epstein-Barr virus. I previously worked in a program with my husband called The Evolved CEO, where we work with high business leaders and CEOs in high-pressure positions. Often, their health was a key area needing focus. Again, it was always linked to EBV. Not a single client through The Evolved CEO business knew anything about EBV, yet 95% had the virus active and causing a lot of mental and physical issues. I also worked with many of The Evolved CEOs' wives, and most had health issues and restrictions due to EBV.

As the business grew, we faced more and more demand, and our fees for working with me increased due to the limited spots available for private work. In the end, I felt really sad because I knew how to heal Epstein-Barr virus, and I knew how much people were suffering in the world today without a solution. I stopped talking about it because every time I mentioned that I knew how to heal it, people would come to me, sad that they couldn't afford my services. So, I worked out a way to create a program and a process that could reach more people and heal more people, specifically for EBV.

I launched this program under my own brand, The Evolved Healer, as I work with many other spiritual healers due to my unique gifts in working with dark energy and dark entities. However, I also find that many healers, even with all their tools, often have issues with Epstein-Barr virus. This is because you have to work with EBV on a multi-dimensional level. It significantly affects a person's physical body, neurological structures, and spiritual connection.

To truly heal EBV and stop it from coming back, you have to work on all levels.

My energetic systems are the template for healing Epstein-Barr virus in others. Over the years, I have developed more skills, increased my gifts, and enhanced my healing abilities. I have story after story, but I don't often share the intricate details of my journey because it has been extremely intense and, at times, doesn't even sound real.

The starting place was Advanced Holistic Kinesiology. I am eternally grateful for this amazing platform.

But now, I don't even know what I would call myself, to be honest with you.

At one point, very early on in my journey, I was told that my teachers would no longer be on Earth and that I would have many guides and teachers over time. This felt so scary to hear at the time. At times in my journey, I felt like I was fumbling in the dark, and sometimes I was.

My biggest development of skills has come through my relationship with dark energies, working at levels that are unheard of, certainly not taught or referenced in books. Reclaiming my power to work at these levels has been challenging. Many times, I have actually worried for my physical safety and life due to the nature of dealing with entities.

I often get asked by other spiritual healers how I've developed all the gifts that I have and how I have these abilities.

Most of the things I do now have not come from books or courses. It was about reclaiming my power within myself, which I didn't know I had at one point.

Developing my ability to command dark energies and entities at the highest levels is what allows me to do the highest light work and spiritual healing possible. Believe me, it has been a major process and journey to claim my gifts and develop my abilities.

At one stage in my journey, my mantra was, "When you're going through hell, don't stop!" To be honest with you, at times, I have wondered if, at the start of my awakening, I had known what I was in for, I might have declined the journey, for it felt unbearable sometimes. I often liken it to opening Pandora's box; once it was open, there was no going back.

I was so shut down, mostly by entity interference. It was a process to remove one thing after another. When I first started working with energetic surrogacy, my first gifts in healing were those of clairsentience.

If you are unsure of what I am referencing, clairsentience is one of the five senses through which a person experiences their intuition.

These five senses are called the "five clairs." They are five different intuitive channels that allow you to receive divine inspiration and messages from spirit.

## Clair #1: Clairvoyance

This is the most well-known of the 5 clairs. Clairvoyance can happen by seeing both internally and externally.

People who have external clairvoyance might see people's auras, energetics as well as multi-dimensional beings and information in the physical world that others cannot.

People who have internal clairvoyance view images or information through their mind's eye; this could be lights, colours, or even full images.

## Clair #2: Clairsentience

This is clear feeling.

This is mainly an internal process. It can feel like heightened emotional and feeling states. It can be almost an extension of "gut feeling," although a person with these gifts can feel things intently, not just for themselves but for others and the world and energy around them.

Empaths and highly sensitive people often experience clairsentience as the ability to deeply perceive and take on other people's feelings and sensations. In these cases, it's important to be mindfully aware of which feelings and sensations are yours and which belong to someone outside of yourself.

This can feel like a burden and often weighs people down, although it is a gift. Gifts can become dysfunctional and all gifts have a positive and negative polarity to them. This sense can become very out of balance for a person.

## Clair #3: Clairaudience

This is clear hearing.

Like clairvoyance, clairaudience can happen both internally and externally.

External clairaudience: this looks like receiving confirmation through a sound medium; maybe it is a phrase in a song on the radio, a person saying something, almost like a message inside a message.

Internal clairaudience: happens when you "hear" messages or words being spoken to you from within.

## Clair #4: Claircognizance

This is clear knowing.

It's a deep sense of certainty, clear knowing in the present moment.

This is an internal knowing that bypasses logic and reason. It comes from a deeper place than memory formation. It's a knowing that arises from deep within, not from your mind.

This can show up as a strong presence within you, simply saying *yes* or *no*. It can also feel like a download of information or new insights, divine knowing that helps you see things from a new perspective.

It resonates at such a deep level within and feels clear, transparent, certain, and deeply true. Claircognizance often requires a lot of trust; trusting fully helps to deepen this sense.

**Clair #5: Clairalience** means "clear smelling." It is the 5th clair and not as common.

These are the main 5 clairs above, although as I looked into expanding my intuition more and more, I heard of another—this clair is almost more like a technique to enhance the others, but it has its own name.

## Clairpretend

This sense uses curiosity and openness to build on your intuition.

It can also serve as a bridge or gateway to activate the other clairs.

It allows us to connect more to free flow energetic and let go of control and the egoic mind that can interfere.

Awakening clairpretend involves asking questions to activate other intuitive abilities. It also leads the way to ask questions that create a clear connection and offer back an intuitive answer.

This is a sense that I did not realise I was using in the process to hear higher information. I would simply ask questions:

- What am I seeing?
- Where am I?
- What do I need to let go of?
- Where does this restriction sit? Are there any other interlinks across mind, body and soul?

These questions are all generally asked in a meditation state, and each question builds on the first and the response that is received back. It involves clearing the mind, releasing expectation and then prompting my intuition as a way to direct it favourably.

I would use this technique to work through old trauma in my energetic bodies and systems.

This sense is always directed by asking open-ended questions to gain more insights and awareness. It is usually done in a curious way. Asking the correct questions can open the mind to receive higher intuitive answers. This is also a skill and ability that can be enhanced over time. It also acts as a gateway for other senses to answer or show you more insights.

Another key piece of information about the spiritual realms and developing intuition, which I have learned over time, is that because we have personal will, we are not allowed to be told what to do. We must direct our consciousness to what we want to create or what answers we are seeking to hear. Intuition is a little tricky because if we are not asking the right question, no answer will come back. Over time, I have learned to reframe my questions to the correct ones, and this has made all the difference.

At the beginning of my journey, with my main sense being clairsentience, I just felt things so intensely. Although, at the time, I did not realise this was a gift, I simply felt sick all the time as entity interference would make me feel this way. Needless to say, I spent years feeling very unwell. At times, it was unbearable.

I remember often looking at other people in my course, those who had obvious gifts like clairvoyance, and feeling disheartened. Why did it feel so hard for me? One day, when I was speaking to another student, I told her I felt as though I didn't have any intuition, and she was shocked. She told me she thought I was one of the most gifted in the whole course. I was confused and said I didn't have any abilities. She then explained that clairsentience was actually an intuitive gift. At this point, this was something I did not understand.

This changed things for me, as I had only seen it as a burden up until then and not useful at all. I often teach people about their intuition and understanding that the way it answers back is a vital part of developing it.

I started developing other gifts at a rapid rate, learning more and more about energy and how to connect, feel, and communicate with it.

Along with being clairsentient and using the framework and learnings I had developed, I also utilised the knowledge I had accumulated over my years of study. Because I used muscle monitoring to get responses, I would use my own muscles as an indication. This was cumbersome and would take me hours to do healing work. I then progressed to almost feeling a shift in my body for a yes or no, and then I started to develop claircognizance, clear knowing.

One of the biggest development tools I used was simply dedication to self. I was in constant fight or flight, dealing with relentless entity issues and having to piece my healing path together bit by bit for myself. I started writing when someone told me about a technique called "ghost-writing," where you clear your mind and write from your higher guidance.

I practised every day. I was desperate to hear my guidance more clearly in hopes of making the journey easier for myself. At first, it was a lot of babble, messages more from the mind that held so many fears and mistruths. But as I got better, I was able to clear my mind long enough to free-write.

I spent months and months, even years, doing this. The messages became clearer, and I was able to clear my mind in a shorter space of time. I got very good at it. It was amazing what this place inside of me would tell me—directing me to heal, offering love, support, and guidance. I progressed even further to writing with other people's guidance, channelling messages. Many beings presented themselves over time to teach me new things. I could write from any energy source, even an animal. If you can interact with energy, it will speak to you.

I channelled for many years; in fact, I have shelves full of journals. Some contain profound insights, new information, and new healing techniques, while others simply document my own trials and tribulations, but always with a focus on healing myself or creating new healing methods to improve my gifts and abilities.

At the end of many chapters, I have included a channelled message from Source, divinity, or guidance—call it what you will. This beautiful guidance always speaks poetically, almost like a poetic remembrance. It is not just thought-provoking but creates an awakening to a heightened level of knowing and truth deep within.

Over time, the channelling turned into clairaudience, where I actually hear things being spoken to me. So, I would be like a medium, but I don't just relay information to people. I use that information to know exactly what I need to do and where I need to heal a person's energetic structures, as well as which body structures are holding stress and why. This is all part of how I heal a person.

At times, this has been a lot to process. I have had to undergo numerous updates in my energy and make changes to my physical body to work in this way.

There is a very fine line between sanity and insanity when it comes to handling the amount of energetic information that comes through your mind at these levels of gifts.

It also takes a lot of mental brain capacity to process energetic information. Once upon a time, even working a few hours would make me tired. Working with two or three people per day took a lot to recover from. But now, as I have trained my energetic system to hold higher and higher frequencies, I can conduct 12 to 15 hours of healing in a day and still function normally, holding hundreds of people's energetics at the same time.

Each time I worked at higher and higher levels, I would have to adapt my body to these new frequencies. Some would have an integration period that could make me very sick until I attuned to this new information and new energetics.

I now work with many multi-dimensional vibrational frequencies that are not of this Earth. They have very high capabilities and healing properties. Over time, I have been shown more and more, although my energetic system had to be capable of holding them. This means it has been a huge progression to even be able to work at these levels.

Since 2017, I have worked privately with hundreds and hundreds of clients on personal healing and transformation. Of these clients, 95%

of them had EBV as the deepest underlying restriction holding them back from optimal mental, physical and spiritual health.

By working at the highest levels of mind, body, and soul, and from working with people's physical bodies, organs, and glands, I was able to create a template for healing. However, as a healer, you must have healed yourself first before you can heal another. My journey to offer the gift of healing to others comes from stepping out of years of health decline. I have spoken about my journey with EBV, with the foundations stemming from the birth of my first daughter, although EBV was active long before that, as I had passed it to all three of my children in utero. My journey to healing encompassed healing myself, my family, and then extending this gift to the world.

## Chapter Summary

In this chapter, I have shared my personal story of struggling with EBV and my health decline, especially after having children. I describe my challenging journey as a mother dealing with my own ill health while caring for my babies. Seeking answers, I turned to many natural therapies including a Chinese herbalist who helped me understand the role of adrenal exhaustion in my condition. Ultimately the deep desire to heal myself set me on a path of intense study and training in Advanced Holistic Kinesiology, through which I developed profound healing abilities and an understanding of the energetic and spiritual dimensions of health. My journey was not easy, as I had to contend with dark energies and entities along the way. However, through dedicated self-healing work, I was able to reverse engineer EBV and develop a powerful healing protocol.

CHAPTER 3

# Mind: How EBV Affects the Brain

The key to understanding Epstein-Barr virus is to recognise that it's an opportunistic virus that uses our body's own stress responses against us.

By now, you'll understand how detrimental Sympathetic Nervous System Dominance (SNSD) is to life and health. However, don't be fooled into thinking that it is simply Epstein-Barr virus that creates this condition. SNSD is already present, and EBV just takes advantage and feeds off this state.

SNSD, also known as compounded deep survival stress, is the perfect feeding ground for EBV to thrive. Many people are overly concerned with trying to control their external stress and toxic environments, overlooking the internal stress response and dysfunction that has been created within themselves.

If I had known how my stress responses worked—and, more importantly, how they were created in the first place—I would have had an opportunity long ago to dismantle them before they co-created with Epstein-Barr virus, taking my health and life to such a vulnerable state. SNSD is predominantly created through the brain being in conflict with itself. It is the conflict between the conscious mind and the unconscious mind that compounds stress.

If I'm honest with myself, my decline began years and years before having children, and the starting place was my own mind. I had so many distorted beliefs about myself, who I was, and the world around me. I lived a life of fear, deep unworthiness, and emotional suppression. My fears wore many faces in my day-to-day life, and it is always those triggers that push us into an unconscious or automatic stress response.

It may look like we grow up, become adults, and learn how to deal with adult problems, but when our brains are still functioning from the fear responses of a child, we are continually stuck in the past, recycling trauma or limiting beliefs over and over again.

These were all things I never took into consideration when dealing with stress or health decline. I often tell my clients that "stress is a lazy word for fear." Especially when it comes to EBV, these stress associations and responses are linked to an energetic memory association with the virus. What I have found over time is that people have their own specific triggers for EBV. In order to heal from EBV, you have to identify, break, and clear these triggers to release the entanglement in the central nervous system so the brain can re-regulate along with the reduction in the virus. This is why one size never fits all when it comes to healing.

EBV is not just a story of disease and ill health; it's a representation of a lifetime of stress.

When we talk about stress, people's conscious minds will instantly associate it with obvious stressors in the present, like a bad day at work, financial stress, or a fight with loved ones. Yes, this is all stress; however, the lifetime of stress that I'm talking about often stems from your childhood, where you may not remember specific events, but all stress holds an unconscious and energetic memory.

So let's dive into how the brain works, how it develops, and discuss circumstances or situations that hold these unconscious stress memories.

Firstly, you need to understand that 95% of our brain's capacity is unconscious and subconscious. This is where stored memories, beliefs, programs, trauma, events, desires, and so much more are kept. The other 5% of our brain's capacity is the conscious mind, where we process our daily thoughts and decisions.

It is very important to understand that we are exposed to millions of bits of information per second every day through all our sensory pathways, including sight, hearing, touch, smell, taste, and energy fields. Our conscious mind has to work out which bits of information are important to process, as the conscious mind can only manage hundreds of bits of information per second and hold up to only seven chunks of information at one time. This helps you understand how easily the mind can be under stress—literally hundreds and thousands of micro-moments per day.

When the mind is constantly under stress (fear), it will draw on past events, feelings, or memories in the unconscious and subconscious mind to form its decision-making. Ultimately, your past negative bias is driving your current decision-making.

Now let's look at how the unconscious and subconscious neural mind is formed and how it draws on stored information, thoughts, and memories that affect our behaviour and decision-making.

When we're born, our conscious brain hasn't developed or come online yet. From ages 0 to 7 is what's called the "imprint period." During this period, the child's brain is like a sponge—everything emotionally significant, both positive and negative, that a child's brain experiences tends to go straight into their subconscious mind. This makes most of the learning during this period subconscious to unconscious.

During the imprint period, kids have not yet developed their mental filters. The most important things to a child are the people who take care of them, protect them, and love them, typically their mother and father.

Another way we form unconscious beliefs and memories is through "mirroring." This means the beliefs, behaviours, words, actions, and energy of our parents, caregivers, and other influential people in our childhood will form our own. So, if your parents were stressed, fought a lot, had money problems, marriage dysfunction, unhealthy habits, and hundreds of other examples, they all become part of your unconscious and subconscious neural pathway programs.

As children, we take on many beliefs from our environment, what we're taught by our parents, friends, families, and school experiences. We absorb all of these programs and unconscious beliefs about our world. These form our early emotional foundations for life and the lens through which we view our world. Often, as a child, the world can be a scary place.

As young children, we all seek these three very important things: Am I safe? Am I loved? Am I worthy?

For many normal, everyday children, their parents pass down a lot of generational trauma and negative beliefs and programs that actually don't serve them.

You don't have to be raised in a dysfunctional, violent, or abusive household to experience childhood trauma. As mentioned before, at the young ages of 0–7, what we seek from our parents is: Am I safe? Am I loved? Am I worthy? Each child's sensory perception of these emotional needs could be different.

For example, parents constantly fighting due to financial stress might make a child feel unsafe hearing those fights. Or a father always working to support the family and not spending any time with the children might make them feel unloved.

These circumstances often get brushed under the carpet, but when you study how the mind works, particularly inner child mind development, you'll learn just how significant those events are in shaping a person's beliefs and programs as they get older.

Now, we move on to brain development between the ages of 7 to 14. Though 90% of the brain has been developed before the age of 7, the brain's complexity becomes the developmental focus in adolescence, as the part of the brain behind the forehead, called the prefrontal cortex, is one of the last parts to mature. This area is responsible for skills like planning, prioritising, and making good decisions. The teen brain is ready to learn, unlearn, and adapt to new experiences and situations. Through these stages of brain development and changes, a child often stops asking their parents, "Am I loved? Am I safe? Am I worthy?" And they start asking the world, friends, and social media, "What do you think of me?" Again, we take on all these compounding beliefs, programs, and thoughts about ourselves as we form our own identity.

It's really important to understand that even though the prefrontal cortex has developed and the adolescent brain thinks it's making its own decisions, this conscious decision-making part of the brain is only 5% of the brain's capacity. The subconscious and unconscious brain make up the other 95%, which was formed and programmed by outside influences, environments, events, and emotional triggers before the age of 7.

So, our identity, behaviour, beliefs, and decision-making are driven by the circumstances that shaped these pre-conscious beliefs and perceptions.

In life, if I haven't examined some of these associations and what I link stress to, it's like I'm running on autopilot. When a situation occurs, the brain's amygdala (flight or fight response centre) initiates an unconscious process that searches my memory bank. It searches the hippocampus for meaning: *What does this event or situation represent? Should I engage a fight-or-flight response or remain calm and safe because everything's fine?* With Epstein-Barr virus, these stress responses, triggers, beliefs, programs, and anchors create the foundation or landscape for the virus to thrive.

At a certain point, EBV uses your stress responses against you. As EBV increases in the body and crosses the blood-brain barrier, inflaming the entire central nervous system, it locks you in stress. It's almost like the chicken and the egg—which came first? Our stress responses play a role, but as EBV heightens in the body, it creates more neurological decline, holding the brain in a state of stress and locking you into Sympathetic Nervous System Dominance. When we are stuck in this state, we lose our ability to heal ourselves, to be in balance, and to regenerate and renew ourselves. This is the pathway to decline.

This is why, when I talk about EBV, I have created a program and a process to look at healing Epstein-Barr virus, examining every single organ and gland in the body, all the neurological structures. You have to consider that Epstein-Barr virus is linked to someone's life, stress responses, and triggers. There will be key times of stress in someone's life that act as foundational blocks for the buildup of Epstein-Barr virus.

When I speak to someone, it's like I can hear or see many of the key restrictions for them that contribute to this constant re-triggering. I see it time and time again: People try to alleviate stress by changing their external lives. They might limit all the things that create stress, but if they haven't healed the deeper reasons their brain associates with stress, and if they haven't cleared that in a healing way at a deep neurological level, any time that situation recurs—and believe me, life happens—they will still be affected. There are many events that come up that might not seem to warrant a huge internal fight-or-flight response, but internally, that's what they create. The key with Epstein-Barr virus is identifying these key moments in your life to find the associations to stress—what allowed Epstein-Barr virus to use your body against you and to build up. In healing these triggers, you must address some of these associations or stress triggers and responses simultaneously because EBV holds an association or an energetic memory attached to all these times. This is why people might do well, reduce it slightly, and then re-trigger it. This re-trigger creates an internal stress response even though it looks like nothing major in their life has happened. We are simply recreating our life from the past.

Epigenetics shows how all past traumas, emotional responses, and our environment shape and change our gene expression. When it comes to healing, you can't just look at someone's current reality.

Often, when people see a healer, they present in deep survival stress, and the healer will take them out of that state.

However, years of Epstein-Barr virus compound into hundreds or thousands of layers of deep survival stress. You may be able to release some of the top layers of stress, but you have to work directly at the level of the virus or find the key triggers of deep survival stress.

This is also known as the web of sub-creation. One moment in time can create the foundation for all other stressful events or associations to continue to feed off or increase from that point. People's stress can be overloaded by the smallest of things. It's really about the brain. The brain is in conflict. Consciously, I might know I'm safe. Consciously, I might want to create whatever it is I aspire to in my life, but it's the unconscious that runs everything.

I would love people to look at their health differently. I would love people to factor in their neurological structures and their mental health because that is the key foundation of health. The brain, neurologically, controls everything else.

You have to regain the ability to access both sides of your autonomic nervous system. You need to be able to return to your parasympathetic state because that is the only place where rest, repair, healing, and cell renewal occur. Life has become so overcomplicated with many pressures and demands. Auto-toxicity is actually the biggest issue. People constantly look at their environment to see what they could eliminate, maybe foods and chemical products. Don't get me wrong: all of those things are important for a foundation of knowledge on health and healing, but it's the auto-toxicity—the internal gauge—that's crucial. Auto-toxicity occurs when we're stuck constantly in that fight-or-flight response, overproducing cortisol, which does significant damage to the body.

People often look at health superficially, focusing on weight gain or aesthetics because they want to look better. But what if mental health was the catalyst and a huge key component in weight gain and other health issues? Because it is. I would love for people to view their health from this higher perspective.

The brain always wants to keep us safe. If it sees something as a threat or danger, it will mount that stress response. We might consciously want to change something in our life, but if we have a negative association or it doesn't feel safe to do that, the brain links this unsafe meaning or a higher stress response to it. We live in a world of overload. If you think about how the brain works, there's so much information it has to process daily, even more so now with the compounding effects of technology. People aren't respecting what is required for good neurological function, what it takes to have a brain that can release stress and manage itself correctly. Our downtime is now spent in front of screens, especially for the next generation. The mind requires silence to heal and repair. The mind needs free space, and most people are getting none in their day.

It's like a computer: Everything I view, everything I see, all this information has to be processed.

I work with a lot of high-level business leaders, teaching them about the nine pillars of success, love, and happiness. The foundational, highest-priority pillars are always health—mental, physical, and spiritual health. Mental health is always number one. I've given talks to companies where people don't understand how their brain works, how it processes all of this information, and how brain overload compounds with unconscious beliefs. Yes, that creates stress, but the modern world, with its constant noise and lack of space, exacerbates this. Technology and other factors contribute to increasing neurological decline.

People often take supplements for their bodies but not for their brains. Even when it comes to elevated consciousness, brain structures need to heal and realign. They have to be capable of holding a higher vibrational frequency and elevated information. When they're stuck in neurological inflammation or stress, it's like we're hindering our own path of progression. So, I would love to ask people, "How much silence do you sit in each day?"

The brain also can't distinguish between what is actually happening and what is not. Many people don't understand the internal gauge of overthinking and not directing their minds favourably. The mind is a tool, but we have to direct it favourably. We either master our mind or become a slave to it. Good mental habits don't just happen; they require the same discipline as creating space for good hygiene, health, or fitness. The mind requires the same discipline.

I see a lot of people exercising, training, or walking, but they have ear pods in or are looking at a screen, adding more information that their brain has to process. I love to talk to people about creating that foundation and space in their daily lives, becoming more aware of how they're looking after their neurological structures. Anything can be a mindfulness practice as long as we're doing one thing at a time. I see many people using technology, looking at two different screens—maybe watching TV while also looking at their phone. That's like splitting, fracturing the mind. I really worry about the next generation, Gen Z and Gen Alpha. This generation has no idea of the compounding effect of neurological overload created by this external world, leading to more internal disconnection and stress.

At one point in my journey, I think I helped a lot of people who didn't realise how their mind was overloaded with energy or constant mind chatter. There's no reprieve, no peace, and perhaps a negative narrative. They're always running scenarios in their heads. I have to talk to my children about this all the time. We can create the same internal stress response as if we're in a stressful situation just by thinking about it. I believe this is something we should be teaching everyone, especially our children: how to manage stress, handle their daily lives, and incorporate these great practices to create space for good neurological function is essential.

The mind always wants to keep us safe, so it either wants to step away from danger or affirm us. Our thought processes are crucial in this regard. When I talk about healing the brain, it's more than just positive thinking; it's about directing your mind favourably. We have something called the Reticular Activating System (RAS), a seeking system, and our brain and mind wants to affirm us. It's like we give it jobs to do; we tell it to seek something out. If I'm always looking at the negative, that's what I will see in my life.

So, when it comes to healing, you have to work at a deep neurological level to release all the stress associations so that the physical body can recover itself. This provides the physical body with a platform for healing and health.

What I learned from completely healing myself from Epstein-Barr virus and mastering the energetic makeup of this virus is that EBV attaches to mercury and crosses the blood-brain barrier. Once it crosses this barrier, it compromises the central nervous system, enabling EBV to seriously deteriorate a person's health into life-threatening illness and disease.

More and more research is coming out linking EBV to neurological diseases such as Alzheimer's and Parkinson's, along with numerous cancers, Multiple Sclerosis (MS), and an incredibly long list of mysterious illnesses.

For most people with highly active EBV, it is significantly compromising their brain, neurological structures, and neurotransmitters. This is why detoxing and restricting your body can be extremely dangerous. A compromised brain, which controls all the automatic functions in the body, can be the very reason you're stuck in Sympathetic Nervous System Dominance, have digestive issues, hormone imbalances, and much more. Detoxing a compromised body can lead to more stress on your systems and allow EBV to take a deeper hold on your health decline.

Stress and brain function, over time, create more and more dysfunction throughout our mind and body. Stress is the number one cause of health decline and disease in this modern world. It is the leading killer and is linked to numerous health issues. It is more important than ever for people to understand their brain, how it functions, and how stress affects us.

Looking back on my life, I wish I had known how my brain worked and how my stress responses had been formed from a very young age. One of the keys to healing is to work directly with the brain to heal our pre-programmed stress responses.

**Chapter Summary**

In this chapter, I have focused on how Epstein-Barr virus affects the brain and creates stress responses that compound the virus's impact on the body. I explained how the unconscious and subconscious mind, formed during childhood, can hold negative beliefs and traumas that fuel stress responses. I also discussed how EBV crosses the blood-brain barrier, inflaming the central nervous system and locking a person into a state of Sympathetic Nervous System Dominance. I have emphasised the importance of healing the brain and unconscious programming to reduce stress triggers associated with EBV. The chapter's primary takeaway is that managing stress properly and understanding how the brain works are crucial for healing.

**Channelled Message** (divine guidance that speaks poetically, awakening a deep, heightened sense of knowing and truth within.)

*In order to facilitate the deepest restorative levels of healing, one must view circumstance correspondingly.*
*The mind, the body*
*Implants, instructional information laying dormant accessible by circumstance.*
*To truly create and recreate self requires many intricate details but at their essence*
*5 principles apply*
*Restore order to the most unruly organ in the body. (The brain)*
*Create new awareness, a mind in deregulation can only multiply this across timelines.*
*A mind with incomplete transition, a mind that occupies the past can never future proof itself.*
*Predators exist across many levels, that pose threat to an already extinct ability – the God-given rights as a self-healing organism.*
*Be wise what truth you recount, for the mind will hold many deviations to a sovereign presence.*
*EBV in all its own variations is interlinked at the level of non-regulation, and is linked into miscommunication. Taking advantage to disrupt networks of structures designed to relay needs, to restore equilibrium.*

*Many years ago your needs changed, and yet this was not reflected in the sacred bonds of natural reordering.*

*Life is Intricate*

*Life is something to hold dearly*

*Instruction, guidance to be nurtured*

*Instruction and guidance to be brought back to life through complete soul recognition.*

*A wavering of self, a slow decline, messages unreceived – this is all interweaved into the energetic associations of a life force eager to reclaim its rights to procreate within itself. (this is talking about the virus)*

*EBV is a standalone virus, but nothing is ever stand alone*

*To dismantle opportunistic layers, one must reverse the opportunity and it is always created through a disconnect so great – The Mind is the breeding ground for a life unlived but the soul, the soul is everlasting and the path trajectory is always to quieten the mind through passing moments, quieten the mind to reorder the physical.*

*Quite the mind and the soul will always speak*

*True mind, body, soul integration is one true identity brought forth into physicality.*

*With this in mind, nothing can deregulate long enough to create the cascade of ill effects.*

## CHAPTER 4

# Body: How EBV Affects the Body

When I was struggling with Epstein-Barr virus at its heightened stages, I felt so disempowered. I would often ask, *What is wrong with me? Why can't I heal myself? What pieces am I missing?* Doctors constantly told me I was depressed, but it didn't feel like depression. It felt like something deeper. I would go through cycles where my life would be manageable, I would be happy, and I would be in alignment. Then, it often seemed to go out of alignment with my ovulation cycles. Before I got my period, I would turn into a completely different person. It was almost like I was Jekyll and Hyde.

It was so confusing because, although I was constantly being told I was depressed, there were times when I didn't feel like a depressed person. There were times when I was handling my life well. There had to be a higher answer. It had to be more related to a hormonal imbalance or other health issues. At that point in time, I didn't really understand how my mind and body worked or how all the different aspects needed to function correctly for optimal health. I remember it being one of my lowest points, and I didn't know what else to do. I ended up posting in a Facebook moms' group.

I was part of a Facebook group called Northern Beaches Mums, where people asked questions about their lives. Maybe I was a little naive, but I kept seeing someone posting really vulnerable comments under the name "Anon." I just thought that was their name and saw them constantly asking questions. Somehow, I thought this was the same person. So, I ended up writing a post and bared my heart to the world. I spoke about being so unhappy, struggling in my day-to-day life, dealing with the demands of motherhood, being a wife, and handling responsibilities and roles that were weighing on me. I felt like there was something deeply wrong. It was almost like a cry for help, but I was also searching for some guidance, some answers as to what I could do to heal and resolve these issues. I posted it under my name. One thing about me is that I've always been very truthful. I tell it how it is, and I don't mind putting myself out there in that way. The feed lit up and blew out of control, with hundreds of people commenting. It was reassuring because many others described their struggles, saying they were in a similar situation and offering advice. I went to my children's school, and people would actually come up to me and say, "Oh my goodness, I can't believe that you wrote that." I had thought Anon was just a person, but Anon means anonymous. One thing I did learn is that there is so much beauty in vulnerability.

I work with a lot of people and am privy to important information about their lives. I feel honoured that people are really vulnerable with me, and I can see that their struggles are also the making of them. I see the points in time when my clients' lives are almost falling apart, like mine was when I posted my vulnerabilities online. We live in a world of social media where people share images and stories of wonderful moments. Yet, we don't know what is really going on for most people.

This is a double-edged sword because most people are struggling mentally, emotionally, and physically. The judgement and comparisons of seeing other people's amazing lives are not a true representation of what's actually happening. People are struggling, and the facade of social media only compounds our struggles and suffering even more.

Being a healer, it blows me away that I meet so many people looking for healing and struggling in many areas of life. However, they look healthy on the outside. Often, you can't actually tell who's healthy and who's not because that external view isn't an accurate reflection of what's happening internally.

I tried for years, and I know I mentioned in my story that the starting place was finding out that I had EBV, but it actually wasn't. If I'm honest with myself, I haven't taken very good care of myself my whole life. I drank a lot of alcohol and masked my emotional pain. I didn't even understand health and what it required to look after myself—mind, body, and soul. My idea of healing was to add more to my daily to-do list, to do another detox, to go to the gym, and to push myself harder. Little did I know all of these things were just compounding my stress deeper and deeper.

When people tell me they're trying all these things and their body isn't responding, I have to explain to them how EBV creates so much more disconnection and stress, how their body's structures aren't functioning correctly, and how heightened stress at a neurological level paves the pathway for more and more decline, allowing EBV to build up over and over.

After posting online, I received a recommendation to see a local Chinese herbalist, which was probably the first time someone took a full holistic assessment of my life. He looked at my commitments, lack of sleep, struggles with babies with colic, lack of family support, and a husband who travelled a lot for work. He basically said he had never seen anyone with more stress than me.

I started taking herbs and supplements to support my adrenals, as I was basically in adrenal burnout. However, what actually gave me some relief was being seen, validated, and told that I was not going crazy or depressed—I was simply in a chronic state of stress. Although I had a long road to recovery, it felt reassuring to know the reasons and that I was not failing as a mother.

I was trying to do all the right things, but I didn't factor in all of my past history. In fact, my children's colic and difficulties as babies came from me. I didn't realise that you pass on your unhealthy gut flora to your unborn baby. So, their foundation for health was my foundation for health, which was a breeding ground for more stress and decline. Even Epstein-Barr virus got passed through in utero.

This journey opened me up to the real impact of chronic stress as I learned new information about healing. I discovered that I was functioning from a deep state of Sympathetic Nervous System Dominance—all new information I had never heard of before.

This is the most important information I first share with everyone when it comes to health, healing, and understanding how EBV thrives in this state and compounds more layers of deep stress until it locks us out of our own natural self-healing abilities. We essentially lose our ability to re-regulate and transition between the sympathetic and parasympathetic nervous systems.

The parasympathetic nervous system is the side of the autonomic nervous system that allows healing and cell repair to occur. Every single cell in the body renews itself within a certain timeframe. Our eye cells renew every 48 hours, stomach cells every four days, skin cells every 30 to 35 days, liver cells every six weeks, and the whole body every seven years.

So, why do disease and illness still exist, and why are they increasing rapidly? The answer lies in being stuck in Sympathetic Nervous System Dominance.

In this state, we overproduce cortisol.

I touched on some of these effects earlier, which include changes to our metabolism, reduced digestive activity, cravings for unhealthy foods, hormonal imbalances, inflammation, low immunity, unhealthy gut flora, toxicity, adrenal fatigue, poor sleep, and much more. In this state, it's virtually impossible for our organs and glands to heal and repair themselves.

Generally, by the time people come to me specifically seeking knowledge about EBV, they find that their health has been in decline for decades. People often think things like food intolerances, digestive disturbances, and hormonal imbalances are all part of getting older. They are not. They are signs of a deeper issue.

We live in a quick-fix, instant-gratification world. Most people are so disconnected and anxious that they're just trying to find the next answer to get by or get ahead, but they're almost always looking externally.

With the vast amount of information in the marketplace, it gets very confusing, especially around health. It can be so confusing that you don't know who to trust.

Even though I've created a way to heal people from Epstein-Barr virus, I understand the pathways through which EBV spreads through our mind, body, and soul. I have the healing gifts and abilities to unwind and heal every level, including each person's past. However, everyone has uniquely different events, circumstances, beliefs, conditioning, and trauma that have allowed EBV to activate and spread throughout the body.

The biggest challenge I see when talking to people about EBV is that the market focuses only on one dimension—the body. However, EBV is a multi-dimensional virus.

So, what are people doing to heal EBV?

## Nutrition

Personally, I have tried many diet protocols and therapies while searching for answers. Nutrition is often the first place people look as they should. This was a big area I focused on before I understood EBV as a multi-dimensional virus.

When I was studying Advanced Holistic Kinesiology and really taking my healing to another level, I realised EBV was the biggest underlying issue of my health decline. I started researching everything on the market about EBV, and like many people, I was led to Medical Medium Anthony Williams' books. People either love or hate Medical Medium. For those who hate him, I think it's really unfair. He is not healing you from EBV; he is simply offering advice on how the virus works and key information about diet and nutrition in his books.

Anthony Williams has exceptional gifts as a medium, but he simply relays information to people and offers teachings on how to reduce the symptoms of EBV through nutrition.

The premise behind nutrition and healing through our diet is that 70% of the immune system is actually in our GI tract. Our digestive system has its own semi-independent nervous system and is the most extensive neural network outside of the central nervous system. This is also known as the "gut-brain."

Your digestive system has a huge effect not just on your physical health but also on your mental health. Ninety per cent of our serotonin, the feel-good hormone, is produced in the GI tract. There's a saying, "Heal your gut, heal your life." While this is essentially correct, the reason why it doesn't work for everyone or takes a very long time is that you would need to be a martyr following an extreme diet, almost like an extended detox. Even then, I've seen people try that, and I don't think it would be enough. As long as you're stuck in Sympathetic Nervous System Dominance, your digestive system will be in a constant state of stress.

As discussed in previous chapters, when we are stuck in Sympathetic Nervous System Dominance, our digestive system will not be in the right state to utilise proteins, fats, vitamins, and minerals correctly. Until you heal deep neurological structures, stress, and imbalance, diet alone will only get you so far. I work with many people who have followed diet protocols and been completely dedicated to trying to heal EBV through diet, but they have lost so much joy, freedom, and the ability to live a normal life. If any diet is followed from a state of fear and helplessness, the diet then becomes another thing causing more neurological stress.

While reading all of Medical Medium's information, I was developing the most profound abilities to access my complete anatomy, physiology, innate intelligence, and energetic matrix level, which enabled me to look at every function, system, and structure in my mind and body. This includes deep brain structures, neurological function, neurotransmitters, all organs, glands, DNA, cellular information, and much more.

Understanding how complex the human body is and understanding every structure, system, and function in the body is like understanding a universe of information.

As I started learning the information that Medical Medium was teaching, I began accessing the energetics of the information and linking this profound information back to my own body. As I healed EBV in my own mind and body at a cellular level, I quickly learned why all the protocols, diets, and therapies were not enough to completely reduce EBV and stop it from ever flaring up again. It was like I was giving my body a list of where to look for EBV, what was happening in my body at a cellular level, where EBV was hiding in my glands and organs, and the dysfunction it was creating in my bodily systems like my thyroid, digestive, autonomic nervous, central nervous, and endocrine systems, and also where it was causing confusion and conflict in my energetic matrix across every level of mind, body, and soul.

Our bodies are amazing self-healing organisms. Given the right support and information, they know how to heal themselves. I was accessing a field of multi-dimensional information as I started to reverse the buildup and heal myself completely of EBV to the point where I learned the natural state that EBV once was before it morphed into what it is today. Now, my energetics hold the template of not only reducing and healing EBV from every gland, organ, system, and cell within my being, but I also learned how to recode the energetics of EBV to stop it from ever reactivating again. Essentially, I cracked the code on EBV at every level and can now heal the virus and return it to its original state, in harmony within my being.

It's important to understand that EBV was not always this dysfunctional and destructive virus. Ninety-five per cent of the world's population has this virus, and humans have had it for generations. However, only recently has EBV morphed into such a destructive virus that is literally killing people. The reason for this is because EBV is symbolic of the world we have created and live in (more on this important information later in the book).

I mastered Epstein-Barr virus on a multi-dimensional level and used my own mind, body, and soul to reverse years of EBV compounding on every level of my being. This means my energy now holds the template for finding and completely healing EBV on a multi-dimensional level, plus recoding the energetic makeup of the virus to stop it from reactivating again.

With this template of information about healing EBV in my energetics, plus the way I heal clients by bringing their energy into my body, I am able to find and read where EBV is in an individual client's mind, body, and soul. This enables me to take them through a process to heal from EBV, just like I healed myself.

This is one of my soul gifts and the reason why I have been able to create one of the most advanced EBV healing program in the world.

I have had many people come to me over the years who had become completely consumed by the process of trying to heal, restricting their diet more and more, adding more and more rules to follow. It feels stifling to not even be able to enjoy some of the simple pleasures that life has to offer.

I had one client who, after years of following endless diet protocols and limiting herself without any success, experienced a profound change and transformation. She was a healer, and most of her issues were entity-related, but the energetic misalignment and stress had caused so much dysfunction in her physical body that she felt completely non-functional, almost as if she were dying.

Her transformation was amazing to watch. Rather than dialling in her health more and more, doing detox and diet protocols one after the other, she found it completely freeing to add back in luxuries like coffee and chocolate, to take part in social events once more, and to actually live her life. You see, her main issue that triggered and heightened the EBV in her mind and body was now cleared, and her body and digestive system were free to re-regulate.

I had another client while I was working in The Evolved CEO transformation program. At that time, I was not solely focusing on Epstein-Barr virus as the key to healing and transformation but was assessing a person's whole life and looking at creating lasting transformation. Most of our clients came for mindset and business growth, but as you will learn after reading this book, no area of life is separate, and everything is interlinked.

This specific client had contracted a parasite in Bali 20 years earlier, which had ruined his life. The most obvious sign was a digestive imbalance, but the discomfort and damage created a knock-on effect in his health decline. He couldn't eat various things without running to the bathroom and could no longer participate in many enjoyable activities in life, especially social events. His diet had become so restricted to avoid a health crisis that could be explosive, embarrassing, and cause days or weeks of pain. Travel created even more stress, and even family holidays had become a source of dread.

He had once been a very carefree person, but he had become almost enslaved within himself. He dreaded travel, his relationships had suffered, and his mindset and outlook on life had deteriorated. These stresses compounded into heightened stress for both his mind and body, resulting in anxiety and, at times, depression.

He had seen specialist after specialist and tried everything to heal his digestive tract. He came for transformation, unaware of the depth of my healing processes. Through the process, I had to heal Epstein-Barr virus, as the years of stress from this incident had created heightened levels in both mind and body, locking him into more and more dysfunction. The digestive system had to be re-regulated via brain structures, reducing EBV in the process and calming the whole central nervous system so the body could adapt, change, and heal itself.

He was absolutely amazed at the process as his digestive issues disappeared, his life expanded, and his confidence and free spirit returned.

I love watching transformations like this because, when it comes to healing, you have to address the deepest underlying issues in the body, resolve the key stress triggers, and always reconnect to yourself and your spiritual aspects.

## Detoxification

Detoxing is another way that people try to eliminate EBV. Detoxification involves cleansing the blood and removing impurities from the liver, where toxins are processed for elimination. The body also eliminates toxins through the kidneys, intestines, lungs, lymphatic system, and skin during a detox.

Generally, detoxing is done through diet and supplementation, limiting food intake with the aid of herbs and tonics. This process frees up more resources so your body can eliminate toxins more effectively.

I was the queen of detoxes. At least two to three times a year, I would put myself through very strict detoxes. At the time, I thought I was doing the right thing, following what I had learned about the benefits of detoxing. I'm glad to see that, over the past ten years or so, there has been a lot more balanced research around the pros and cons of detoxing and why it's not for everyone, as everyone's health circumstances are unique.

It's vital to be aware that using detoxes for EBV could be the worst thing you could do for your body. Here is why:

Epstein-Barr virus affects your liver detoxification pathways. When these are not functioning correctly, people can actually do more damage by doing a liver detox because they mobilise all the toxins in their body, but the pathways to remove them are blocked, pushing the toxins back into circulation instead of releasing them, which ultimately can do more damage.

This is why so many people, especially women, who try to lose weight simply cannot remove the fat from stubborn areas like the belly, hips, and legs. The body has stored all these toxins in the fat tissue.

When your body doesn't want to release the toxins from your fat cells, it's because it doesn't have the resources to process toxins correctly.

At one stage of my journey, I went on a strict detox weight loss diet to try to remove fat from my hips and waist. However, I lost weight from my chest and breasts, which made me feel so low.

This was before I understood what I am sharing with you now. My body was simply protecting itself from years of toxicity as it didn't have the resources to help balance out my stubborn areas where fat was stored.

If you are going to detox, you need to use a binder to help bind the toxins and aid their passage through the body.

Epstein-Barr virus specifically affects the methylation of liver detoxification pathways. This pathway plays a significant role in processing hormones, so when it's compromised, our hormonal balance is thrown out. On my journey to find healing answers, I was constantly told I was a poor methylator, meaning my body didn't process hormones properly.

This led to significant hormonal and emotional trauma and imbalance. The solution offered to me was a supplement, and one doctor even tried to prescribe me antidepressants. This is a sad reality for millions of women around the world who are experiencing what I did.

As I tracked Epstein-Barr virus in the body, I realised that EBV also attaches to mercury. As discussed in previous chapters, this is a key to understanding how EBV affects the mind and body. To reduce EBV, you must reduce mercury because this is how it crosses the blood-brain barrier to inflame and attack the central nervous system. Mercury, being a neurotoxin, can confuse your body into thinking that it doesn't have enough of it. This causes the body to either not release it or continue to absorb it from other sources.

Not all toxin binders are equally effective, which is why I have sourced one of the highest-quality Zeolite products in the world directly from the manufacturer in Australia. Zeolite is a crystalline mineral compound that cages and removes toxins, helping the body eliminate toxins. More importantly, when my clients purchase this toxin binder, I also code the energetic makeup of the product to hold energetic information about Epstein-Barr virus, mercury release, and instructions to clear any neurological confusion related to this neurotoxin, enhancing the product's healing abilities and effectiveness.

The lymphatic system is another critical area of the body when it comes to healing from EBV. Our lymphatic system, if you don't know, is our body's waste management system, and if it is not functioning correctly, it makes healing extremely challenging.

The lymphatic system is part of the immune system. It is designed to fight off infections, bacteria, viruses, and parasites. It removes toxicity from the body and cleans all the fluid in our body, reducing inflammation and fluid retention. You can actually see when someone has an unhealthy lymphatic system—they will look puffy, inflamed, and retain a lot of fluid.

Ways to maintain a healthy lymphatic system include exercise and movement. Hydration is obviously a really big one. Rebounding on a mini trampoline is also effective. You can get a mini tramp at home because bouncing on it regularly, even for short periods, is one of the best exercises you can do for your lymphatic system.

Additionally, you can do this in a swimming pool. If you jump up and down or do aqua jogging in a pool, it also benefits your lymphatic system. The added benefit of the compression of the water and the cooling of the body temperature makes it even more effective.

Lymphatic massage is another important way to support the function of the lymphatic system. You can see a specific lymphatic massage therapist, or there are really easy techniques that you can learn and practise on yourself.

Supplements are a big factor that people consider. However, you can be dehydrated at a cellular level, which will affect the uptake of different vitamins, minerals, and amino acids. Neurologically, there can be reasons why your body is not able to utilise these nutrients. If there are neurological interplays or restrictions, the body simply won't use the supplements if it doesn't think it needs to. There can be a deeper reason behind the need for supplements, and often, supplementation might seem ineffective because if your body can't utilise them properly, they might just go to waste. Epstein-Barr virus affects the entire digestive system and contributes to dehydration and other issues, so supplements might not address all the compromised areas.

## Energy Healing

When our energy is balanced and aligned, we have an amazing ability to self-heal. But you need to be able to work at the root cause. Often, when you see an energy healer or someone doing healing work, you will present in a state of stress. Most healers simply work on the top layer or the current level of stress. Epstein-Barr virus compounds years of stress and holds the memory of past stress events, so you would need to release hundreds of layers to get to the root cause.

Unless you have a healer who can actually direct your energy, look at specific structures, and know where EBV is and where it's compromised, it can be really hard to address it. EBV can hide in the body, so you need to work at the root cause, not just the symptoms of adrenal or thyroid issues. You have to address the deepest underlying cause when it comes to healing.

The problem I see time and time again is that people have done healing to reduce the virus, but it builds back up again when they're dealing with another stressful event or time.

I have to work at the deepest levels within a person's neurological structures, organs, glands, body systems, and at a soul and spiritual level because they are all interconnected in who and why each person has been compromised by EBV.

This is why, when it comes to healing Epstein-Barr virus, one size doesn't fit all. You have to understand the role our neurological structures play in regulating our body and our health, and also how the body compensates for itself over and over again.

For most people, by the time they're aware of an issue with EBV, it is long-standing and deeply embedded in many aspects of their mind, body, and soul.

The modern world is full of noise, judgement, and comparison, leading us to push through almost everything as a way to survive or get ahead. This results in most people ignoring the signs and symptoms their bodies are showing them.

When we ignore these signs and symptoms or push them down, we compound unhealthy stress and exacerbate EBV over time. It's almost like we've been programmed to push ourselves to a tipping point, like a bucket that is so full it starts to overflow. Once we reach these tipping points and overflow stages, we have a lot of work to do to unwind and heal, often requiring a lifetime of healing.

In the past, people might have had more resilience and been able to handle stress better, or at least thought they could. However, as life goes on and we do not heal and deal with unresolved internal conflicts and health issues, the imbalance and EBV compounds.

It's like we tip over and lose our baseline. We lose resilience because our internal gauge has become so inflamed, pushing us further into stress, decline, illness, and eventually disease.

## Adrenal Dysfunction

When it comes to health, understanding adrenal dysfunction is crucial. All the clients I see come to me with some form of adrenal dysfunction, many of them in the later stages due to EBV.

Adrenal dysfunction has three stages:

## Stage 1: Adrenal Fatigue

This is when signs and symptoms occur. We've overdone it, and our adrenals signal us with feelings of tiredness, fatigue, and flu-like symptoms. It's our body's way of signalling to slow down and rest. However, most people, especially those with many demands, ignore these signs and try to stimulate themselves to create energy. Stress is a form of stimulation that produces more cortisol and adrenaline, as are caffeine and energy drinks.

We overproduce cortisol, which is a steroid hormone that masks many signs and symptoms our body shows us until we push ourselves into the next stage of adrenal dysfunction.

## Stage 2: Adrenal Exhaustion

When we enter adrenal exhaustion, we might feel like we have more energy and that we're handling life and its demands better, but this is deceptive. It's false energy, and it will eventually run out, causing us to deteriorate underneath. This is why many people living in a state of adrenal exhaustion get sick when they go on holiday. These are signs that you have been in adrenal exhaustion, and your body is simply trying to re-regulate itself by moving back into adrenal fatigue, asking you to slow down, rest, and repair.

I was in adrenal exhaustion for years, dealing with kids not sleeping, sleep deprivation, the demands of three children, running a home, a husband travelling all the time, and no family around me to lean on. I felt like I had no choice. I was seriously in adrenal exhaustion. The less sleep I got and the more demands I had, the more I felt like I was handling things better. But the truth is, if I had stopped for too long, I would have fallen apart. This leads me to the next stage of adrenal dysfunction.

## Stage 3: Adrenal Burnout

This is the place of complete mental and emotional breakdown. I've been there, and it's very hard to recover from, especially if you don't make significant changes in your life. Having been to this level, I would not wish it upon anyone. Your body literally cannot keep overproducing cortisol at those levels. It has no more reserves to draw on. Epstein-Barr virus has a massive interplay with these levels of decline. You get pushed further and further into adrenal dysfunction. It's really important for people to understand these stages and become more aware and disciplined around balancing rest and repair. However, as the world speeds up, people are living their lives in these robotic states.

When clients come to me, many are proud to say, "I never get sick." This is often not a good sign if you have been in adrenal dysfunction for a long time. You should probably get sick once or twice a year. It's how our body updates itself through the virome.

My mum once gave me a book called *Rushing Woman's Syndrome* by Dr. Libby Weaver. It was full of great information about the world we live in, about demands, and about managing our minds. But it also said, "Don't be a rushing woman and skip right to the end of this book for the conclusion or the real key pieces of information you need to know."

I have to admit, I skipped to the end of the book. I was the rushing woman. And I think that when it comes to health and healing, we need to reassess our lives. We need to look at health on a deeper level because Epstein-Barr virus affects all levels of a person's being.

It's not just health concerns that you're looking at; it's the history of those health concerns that you need to consider. It's important to not simply focus on your current symptoms but instead look at your history, your past, and key moments in your life where trauma has occurred. These moments may be the catalyst for understanding when EBV first truly activated for you.

## Chapter Summary

In this chapter, I explained how EBV affects the physical body and the importance of understanding the role of the autonomic nervous system in health and healing. I shared my personal struggles with adrenal dysfunction and the stages of adrenal fatigue, exhaustion, and burnout. I discussed how being stuck in Sympathetic Nervous System Dominance prevents the body from healing and repairing itself and how EBV exacerbates this condition. I introduced various approaches to healing, including nutrition, detoxification, and energy healing, emphasising the importance of addressing the root cause of EBV rather than just the symptoms. I also highlighted the connection between the liver, methylation pathways, and hormonal imbalances in relation to EBV.

CHAPTER 5

# Spirit: Vibrational Frequencies and Energy

Before I started on my healing journey, I didn't understand that I was a spiritual being. I had heard the word soul used, and of course, everybody has a soul, but what did that really mean? How was it part of me? Which parts were it? How would spiritual healing or soul healing make a difference in optimising my physical health or happiness?

In the search for reconnection, health, and happiness, a lot of the modalities or techniques I turned to were alternative therapies. It wasn't until I started studying Advanced Holistic Kinesiology that I began to understand more and opened myself to what was possible. It fascinated me, this place that exists within all of us—our soul aspects: how it holds a template, something called our innate intelligence, wisdom so great that if it is given a chance to speak, it will guide us on the correct path and back home to ourselves.

This, for me, was the biggest journey of all: reconnecting to my spiritual aspects and healing my soul. If there is one thing I want you to understand from this book, it is that we are souls having a human experience, and our purpose for being here in this lifetime is simply to grow, evolve, and experience the true essence of our soul, our soul's gifts, and our soul's purpose.

Throughout this book, I talk about how EBV and other blocks and restrictions affect our mind, body, energy, and spiritual connection. These are all interconnected, and we must heal and align all areas and dimensions to fully access our soul's highest potential.

Our body is the gateway to our spiritual and soul aspects, so when we have heightened or compounded EBV built up in our mind and body, it creates blocks, restrictions and disconnection to these higher spiritual and soul aspects.

This deep disconnection not only causes health issues but also causes a deep aching at the level of our soul. We are always longing and needing to come back into balance with all aspects of who we are in mind, body, and soul.

I've seen Epstein-Barr virus as a large contributor to holding people back from their soul's gifts and spiritual connection. It literally felt like they were living in an endless cycle of the dark night of the soul.

## What Is the Dark Night of the Soul?

The dark night of the soul refers to a condition in which people get locked out of their connection. It's meant to be a transition stage to elevation, and going through a dark night of the soul should and can help a person unlock new gifts and parts of themselves. However, Epstein-Barr virus can seriously interfere with this process.

Everyone has a "soul divine blueprint," an energetic template that holds so much information and wisdom, not only about this lifetime but all past lifetimes. It holds our highest potential but, unfortunately, can also hold a lot of restrictions.

To experience higher levels of our soul, purpose, and gifts, we need to work on all levels of ourselves simultaneously!

It's extremely important to understand that we are multi-dimensional beings, existing in all the following dimensions (which are explored in more detail throughout the chapters):

- **First Dimension (1D):** Earth's Core.
- **Second Dimension (2D):** Telluric realm. This is the intricate internal workings of the earth's diverse internal landscape, including chemicals, minerals and microorganisms. It is also home to viruses and parasites.
- **Third Dimension (3D):** The physical world, including your physical body and every other structure you see: trees, animals, cars, houses—literally everything in the physical world
- **Fourth Dimension (4D):** This is the level of the mind, thoughts, Wi-Fi, radio frequency; this also includes the collective and the level of duality.
- **Fifth Dimension (5D):** The start of your spiritual and soul aspects.
- **Sixth Dimension (6D):** From a human aspect, this is when we are living in alignment with our divinity and actioning this into the world.

When it comes to higher dimensions, there are books written about the tenth through to the thirteenth dimensions, but I can tell you there are hundreds of dimensions as I work in them. In a later chapter on entities, I explain more about why I have been granted the ability to access dimensions in the hundreds.

## Let's Talk About Energy and Why It Is So Important for Healing

Everything in the universe is made of energy. Matter is made up of atoms, and quantum physicists have discovered that physical atoms are made up of vortexes of energy that are constantly spinning and vibrating, each radiating its own unique energy signature.

Vibration and frequency are the languages of the universe. It's how the universe works. This is why healing is so important.

As we raise our energetic vibration, we attract higher-quality things to us, including more harmony and balance. The universe doesn't judge us; it simply mirrors back the energy we exert, like what we're putting out, along with reading our soul vibration rate and all our energetic information.

When we elevate our frequency, we attract higher-quality things, as like attracts like. But what is very important to understand is that we can't only focus on the spiritual or the quantum and ignore all other dimensions, as we are multi-dimensional beings. It's important to understand the interplay between all dimensions, energy, vibrations and supports.

## Vibrational Support

Everything vibrates at a certain frequency, even our thoughts and feelings. For example, love has a vibrational frequency of 528 megahertz. All human emotions have a frequency, with negative emotions like guilt and shame holding the lowest frequencies and love, joy, and peace holding the highest frequencies.

If our thoughts, feelings, and emotions all have a vibrational frequency, so do all the body's organs and glands. Each carries its own unique energy.

For instance, a liver vibrates at a different frequency than a heart. Even different brain structures have a vibrational frequency. When I do healing work for anyone, it's like I'm reading these energetic vibrations or frequencies, and often they're out of balance. They're not even vibrating at the right frequency. So, when I harmonise someone's energy and bring it back into balance, it promotes the body's ability to increase its own healing and repair.

We're energetic beings. The human body has an electromagnetic field, so even external energies can affect our energy bodies. The more balanced and aligned someone's energy is, the better their health will be. Different frequencies hold different healing abilities, power, and information.

This diagram shows the different emotional vibrational frequencies of different states of being, whether you are suffering, getting by or in flow.

Fear, shame, and guilt hold lower vibrational frequencies, which will contract your energy, whereas love and joy hold higher vibrational frequencies, which will expand your energy. We all know how good it feels when we're experiencing those elated, expanded states and feelings.

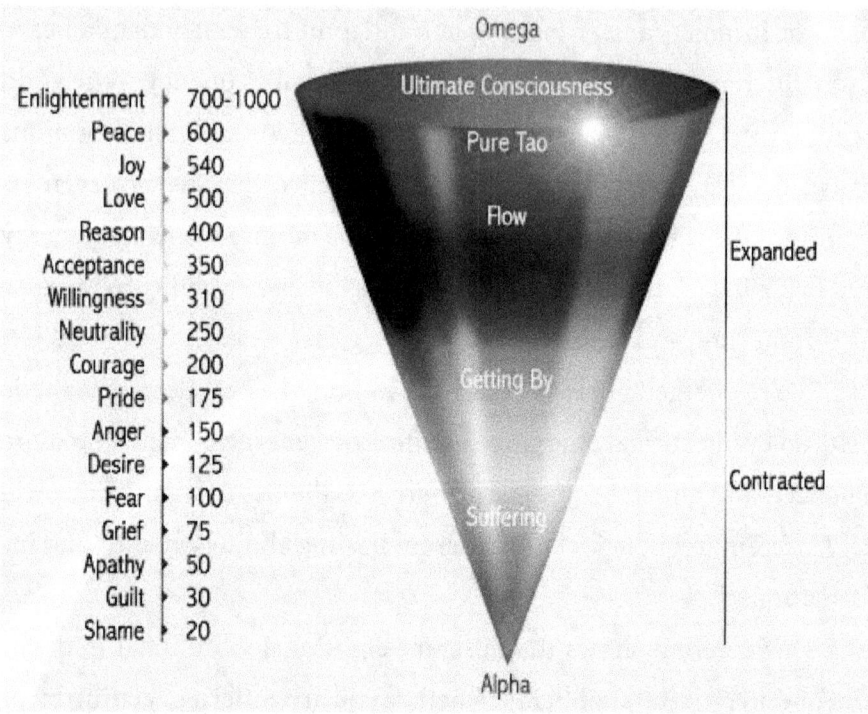

As we understand how thoughts, emotions, and feelings have their own vibrational frequencies, it's important to understand that healing-anchored emotions, beliefs, and trauma from our past are also important parts of healing EBV and expanding our health and well-being.

Earth's energy, **the first dimension (1D)**: You may be familiar with this information, but Mother Earth's natural heartbeat rhythm is a frequency of 7.83 hertz, also known as the Schumann resonance. Mother Earth is designed to take our mental state and replenish us. When you go on holiday, you might notice people feel really energised and great, like when we're at the beach and barefoot on the Earth. It's because we're interacting with this energy that helps to support and heal us. That low vibrational frequency resonates with our cells' vibrational frequencies. There's even a full healing modality called grounding, which talks about the science behind tuning in to the Earth. It helps to reduce EMF radiation.

So, my question is, how often are you connected to the Earth?

We can become really disconnected without realising it. From wearing shoes all day, staying inside, and rarely interacting with this beautiful Earth energy that's meant to support, heal, and nurture us.

The Earth's energetic vibration is shifting, and we're being asked to shift with her. There are many changes in the Earth at the moment. The Schumann resonance can change at different times, and we're all being called to heal ourselves and go through an awakening process.

There's no better time than now to do this healing and alignment work because humanity needs to evolve and change in alignment with the world's and Earth's energetic shifts.

The challenge is that physically connecting with the Earth is not enough these days. As multi-dimensional beings, we need to be connected and aligned on all dimensions, from Earth frequencies to the highest spiritual and multi-dimensional energetic frequencies. I'm seeing more and more people struggling and suffering with these shifts and feeling more and more out of balance, regardless of the effort and healing work they have been doing.

The physical realm is only about one-tenth of what truly exists, what we can see with the naked eye is so very limited. We are actually only 10% Human; there are many other books written on this fascinating topic. This is why it's important to understand the Telluric realm, **the second dimension (2D)** because this is where EBV sits; it is the realm of parasites, viruses, microorganisms, as well as the intricate life forms and elements deep within the earth, it's critical to heal and balance this dimensions if you want to heal from EBV.

EBV is creating more and more spiritual decline, resulting in more mental and physical imbalance and disharmony, and in turn, the physical imbalances and dysfunction are creating more and more spiritual disconnection

Our body is the gateway to the spiritual, so when we have years of restrictions and imbalance in our organs and glands, including our neurological brain structures, it creates a disconnection from our spiritual aspects. For our brain to hold higher states of elevated consciousness, our brain structures need to be able to handle that new information or frequency. They need to be restored and elevated to be able to connect at this higher level.

People often say to me that they want to be more spiritually intuitive, and I ask, "Are you listening to your body?" It's as if our body has been showing us signs and symptoms of decline, fatigue, and stress for a very long time, yet we ignore it. The thing is, messages and intuition come through our body—it's called body wisdom. The clearer we are in our energy, and the more in tune we are with ourselves, the better we know what is right for us. We stop seeking answers externally and start to listen within.

A great example of this is when someone is pregnant.

When I was pregnant, there were different things I craved. But with my last child, I suddenly started craving and eating copious amounts of licorice, even though I didn't like licorice. I was also really struggling with my health, feeling fatigued and tired. When I went to the doctor, I found out I had really low blood pressure. I asked the doctor for natural alternatives to help raise my blood pressure, and they said, "Licorice." I was already naturally gravitating towards it.

When we are clearer in our energy and listen to our body, we receive responses that are almost like signals. Even our emotional body—our emotions and feelings, are gateways to transformation. People often push hard and uncomfortable emotions down to avoid them because they think mental health is simply negative thoughts or emotions. However, thoughts, emotion and feeling trigger responses in our body, leading to a physical reaction. Different structures engage or disengage, fight-or-flight responses happen, and neurotransmitters are involved—there's a physical response to these feeling states.

I love the analogy of the oyster and the pearl. The pearl starts off as a grain of sand, which constantly causes irritation. As the oyster secretes substances to manage this irritation, it eventually turns into something really beautiful. This is symbolic of our emotions and feelings. We need to be listening. We're receiving guidance all the time, but many people look to the spiritual as if it's outside of them. I see this often: They're looking for confirmation and external signs, which is actually a paradigm called superstition. Superstition is when people see a black cat and think it means bad luck. We're actually receiving internal signals, and when the body gets so blocked and restricted by EBV, this then creates a more spiritual disconnection.

The spiritual holds a template for the physical and helps restore and reorder it. There are different orders when it comes to the spiritual and the physical, and they are called positive space-time and negative space-time. The natural balance of the spiritual is for things to be in order. However, in the physical world, **the third dimension (3D)**, everything is physical and solid, and we are separate, and the natural balance is disorder. It's like your house—the big mess.

It just seems to get messier and messier, and you have to put effort and energy into tidying it up. It's the same with these orders. The more we tune in to the spiritual and reconnect, the more we access this beautiful place of higher wisdom, intelligence, to bring reconnection and order to the physical.

At the level of someone's higher self, their soul aspects hold a beautiful thing called their innate intelligence. This is the place I connect to when doing healing work for someone. Their higher soul aspects know exactly what they require to achieve optimal physical, mental, emotional, and spiritual health. The more connected we are, the more aligned and balanced we are in our energetics, and the more this reflects in our physical well-being and health.

**The fourth dimension (4D)** is the level of the mind. We can't see these frequencies, but they exist—thoughts and similar phenomena.

To explain a little bit more about energy and its importance, there's so much energy, and we're always engaging with it. As discussed previously, Earth is one source of energy. Mother Earth's natural heartbeat rhythm is the frequency of 7.83 Hz, known as the Schumann resonance. The 7.83 Hz frequency is an alpha-theta brainwave frequency in the human brain, which is associated with a relaxed, dreamy sleep state when cell regeneration occurs. It is no surprise that people nowadays, especially in bigger cities, are unbalanced, irritated, reactive, angry, and experiencing rising rates of disease.

We live in a time of technology with superficial wavelengths that disrupt the natural Earth's frequency. Wi-Fi, cell phones, and an array of electromagnetics are part of our everyday lives. This is why our bio-electromagnetic waves are out of balance. We are out of balance with the Earth's electromagnetic frequency. For example, the frequency of

5G, radio frequency, and electromagnetic radiation, which power cell phones, TVs, and radios, ranges from 30,000 hertz to 300 billion hertz. That is significantly more than the 7.83 Hertz that the Earth radiates. No wonder we are out of balance and craving healing. We're engaging with different energies all the time.

**The fifth dimension (5D)** is the start of someone's spiritual aspects. It is in alignment with your heart space and the natural world. From there, it extends to our higher soul aspects. At the level of our heart space and spiritual aspects, it works via intention.

We have to be really intentional to create our life.

An intention is a direct focus of consciousness on what we want to create. People who are disconnected and in ill health often stop looking at creation with a positive intention and become so overrun that they almost can't help but see all the negatives.

Before they realise it, their focus and intentions are on ill health, suffering, and even depression and anxiety, making them feel even more helpless and stuck.

There is immense power in looking at things from a perspective of positive creation, but this requires focus, willpower, discipline, and the right healing and support systems to guide people through their journey.

## There are three types of energy: Jing, Qi, and Shen energy.

Jing energy is our body's reserves; it's like our primal energy, it is stored in our kidneys. We have a finite amount, so when our Jing runs out, that's the end of our life. Many people live their lives by continuously drawing down on their body energetics, depleting themselves.

Qi energy is well-known. It's almost like the pathways in the body. We can build this up. The energy of the Earth, the Qi, is strongest first thing in the morning. Running pathways in the body, exercise, movement, and breathing—all these activities create a buildup or extension of Qi. If we build up our Qi first thing in the morning, it's like we're drawing on different energetics. Once that runs out, we'll revert to our Jing, our body reserves.

And then there's Shen energy, probably the most exciting. This is spiritual energy. When we are really reconnected to our spiritual aspects—the divine, call it what you like—it reflects in our health and almost gives us a higher energetic source.

So, you need to understand the truth of elevated consciousness. When my brain is held and stuck in a deep survival stress state, it cannot attune to these higher elevated states of consciousness. Higher elevated states of consciousness involve higher frequency, higher energetics, higher wisdom, and higher information. The more I attune to this elevated consciousness, the more I see a bigger picture. I move out of low-level energetics, fear, depletion, and other negative states, which in turn contributes to longevity, health, and my body holding the right instructions and information for health and well-being. Our neurological pathways need to update to expand and elevate our consciousness; otherwise, they remain stuck in low frequency or decline.

This is how Epstein-Barr virus creates so much spiritual decline. It is nearly impossible to elevate and heal brain structures with heightened levels of EBV, causing more and more neurological decline and disconnection.

The universe does not judge us; it mirrors back what we put out. Vibration is everything, and we each have our own vibration, which is called a "soul vibration rate." When someone's soul vibration rate is between 4 and 4.9, their higher self functions from the same place as their mind and ego, making it hard to distinguish higher guidance from mere mind noise and fear-based programs. But when someone's soul vibration rate is from 5 to 5.9, they shift from the fourth dimension to the fifth, marking the start of their spiritual journey.

There is a proverb that says, "The longest journey someone will ever make is from their head to their heart." When we start living from this higher place, we raise our energetics and realise we are more than just our minds. We also take more responsibility for all that we have created. Regardless of whether we know it or not, we choose all these things in our lives. When we incarnate, we set up all these situations. Many people ask, "Why am I suffering? Why do I have these issues?" Most people's lessons come through suffering; it's how the soul learns. By examining these stories and beliefs that we have carried for so long—beliefs that may not even belong to us—we undergo a process of elimination. Up to a certain point, we absorb beliefs and programs like a sponge, and then we need to reprogram ourselves. We start to question what is true and what is not: "Someone said this about me. Someone said that."

Then, we start to question whether those beliefs are actually right. We begin to discard the beliefs, limitations, and fears we've been carrying. We start to live in greater alignment with our truth and our divinity, **the sixth dimension (6D)**, which is the essence of who we are at a higher soul level. That's our purpose here. The fifth dimension (5D) represents self-discovery; it's called spiritual awakening. Many people, in their day-to-day lives, feel a missing connection to themselves, regardless of what they're searching for. The answers are always within, at the soul level, but the soul's voice is quiet. Soul desires are like whispers, while ego desires are loud. This quietness is due to our free will; we are not allowed to be told what to do.

This is why intentions are so important. We must direct our consciousness toward what we want to create. I love the saying, "The unexamined life is not worth living." When it comes to spiritual guidance, many people don't understand how it works. We can't be told what to do.

We have to direct our consciousness favourably towards what we want to create, and then we receive guidance and support to show if it's aligned. However, we also need to ask the right questions. Many people ask, "Why is this happening to me? What have I done wrong?" When engaging with the spiritual, as I do, if you don't ask the right questions, you don't get a response. If I do healing work for a person and ask a question but receive no answer, it means I've asked it the wrong way. I have to reframe it. Many people try to create from negative intent, which is knowing what they don't want. I understand that the world is in decline and that people are suffering—I see it all the time. But the key to unlocking suffering is to go through it. It involves examining the stories, representations, and reasons for its existence, as there is learning, evolution, and growth in all things.

We have spiritual guidance, but we can also have dysfunctional guidance. When I heal people, these are the things I help release. Dysfunctional guidance involves taking on spiritual guidance, most of which comes when we are children. As children, we don't have many choices available to us, and emotionally, things can feel overwhelming. We may struggle to deal with situations because we lack life experience, emotional sensibility, or emotional control. We learn these skills over time. However, if we find ourselves in situations where we must go against our divinity, the truth of who we are, we may adopt a guide that runs a program or coping mechanism for us.

I see people wanting to step out of limited ways of being or long-standing patterns and often, they have guides running these programs. These guides are not negative; they have been doing a job for us, supporting us in the ways we need. But when people seek to make significant changes or paradigm shifts, essentially changing their destiny, their spiritual guidance must update accordingly.

I see people doing endless healing work in the spiritual realm, and it can become a never-ending process where one can get lost. Initially, spirituality is exciting and fun, but it can lead to feeling lost.

When it comes to healing, especially if people start diving into past lifetimes, we've had so many. Regarding EBV, everyone needs to identify, heal, and release past events, beliefs, and programs that caused the highest activation, creating an energetic tie to EBV reactivating repeatedly.

These events can also be generational at the DNA level, involve epigenetics, and have links to past lifetimes. When you start diving into past lives, the information is endless, and not all of it is relevant to this life. This is where people continually work on issues repeatedly, potentially creating programs that supersede restrictions at the Akashic record or unconscious belief level.

This is why I also help people who get stuck in healing cycles, seeing one healer after another without ever reaching the true, deepest underlying cause of their ill health and disconnection.

Programs can overarch other issues. Remember, the universe doesn't judge us; it mirrors back what we put out. We can create energetic rules, programs, and new agreements to work on all lifetimes simultaneously. This can make the work endless and lead to a lot of unnecessary suffering. I know this because I did it, and I would not wish it upon anyone. With many clients, especially people who have done a lot of spiritual work, I can change these programs for them and free them from the relentless and endless healing cycles.

People often get curious about their past lifetimes, wanting to know every detail, but this can be a distraction. You don't need all the details; all you need is to identify the key pieces from past lifetimes that are present in this lifetime. It is about looking at your current life. When it comes to Epstein-Barr virus, certain key pieces or triggers will have initiated the virus's buildup. Remember, EBV is an opportunistic virus. It uses your stress responses against you, exploiting the conflict between your unconscious and conscious mind and between your ego and your soul. We always strive to come back into balance with ourselves, which is what we are here to do. The soul will keep recreating situations to harmonise itself. Asking, *Why is this happening to me?* is not helpful because there is always a reason. What we don't heal, we repeat. That's how it works.

Finding the key information for healing EBV is crucial. When people come to me for EBV healing, I emphasise transformation. It's like coming home to yourself, harmonising your ego with your soul's potential, and aligning what we're here to do—harmonising our genetic integrity with our soul's potential. In this lifetime, we've agreed on the lessons we want to learn. We set up these situations with other souls, soul groups, family dynamics, and relationships to play out the scenarios that provide our biggest lessons. This is why reflecting on your life and history is so important; the keys to transformation are within this lifetime. By enhancing this lifetime, you enhance them all. I also do a lot of soul retrieval for people.

Our soul is so big we don't actually have access to all of it, and there are two reasons for this. One is the need to heal and resolve trauma. As we resolve our trauma and karma, we get to reclaim these pieces. It's almost like being locked out of it, or it has fractured over time. The other reason is that we may not be ready for the directive of our soul yet. I might not be the person who could even facilitate that new soul's directive because my vibrational frequency isn't at the necessary level.

Such untapped potential and unclaimed gifts are significant. Sometimes people think there is only one fate or one destiny, but there is not. It's called a "paradigm shift." Through working with people, I might facilitate 30 or 40 paradigm shifts over the course of, say, a six-month program. This is essentially changing someone's destiny. It's like elevating them in alignment with their soul blueprint; there's always more to step into.

## The Liver and Transformation

Our liver plays a huge role in transformation. The liver is one of the first places where EBV will settle, affect, wait, and feed off toxicity. From this place, it builds up. But the liver is about more than just physical transformation; it is crucial for spiritual reconnection. The liver's time is between 1 a.m. and 3 a.m., and during this period, it performs many updates. This is also the time when we reconnect with our spiritual guidance, making it the most spiritually significant time of the day. It is linked to brain chemistry replenishing because our brain needs to hold higher vibrational frequency and elevated consciousness. However, many people today do not understand this. Even alcohol disrupts this process because it gives the liver another job to do on top of its existing ones.

I drink alcohol at times, but once upon a time, it was my suppression mechanism. It was how I dealt with life to dull myself down. I didn't realise the compounding effect it had on my physical health and, more importantly, on my spiritual disconnection. Now, I drink occasionally, but my spiritual time at night—that reconnection—is so important that I wouldn't do anything to disrupt it.

Our connection is sacred. It's a sacred relationship that requires dedication and time. Many people are not making time for it. Even in the times when I have extended myself the most, I often get asked by healers how I developed my gifts. My pathway to do this was through soul expansion and soul growth, partly due to my journey with dark entities and dark energies, which I discuss in the next chapter. But when things got really hard for me, I just kept coming back to myself. Because my gifts were unique, I didn't have a roadmap provided by someone else; the roadmap existed within me. I even help many healers, and I'm amazed at how many are not doing the work for themselves. We live in a world of quick fixes—take a pill, do this, do that. But even your spiritual guidance, when people say they want to be more intuitive, requires time.

I teach people how to really reconnect with their guidance. Many don't even know how their energetic systems work, so how can they recognise the response when it comes? It's like a relationship where you have to invest time and get to know it. I also see people approaching their spiritual guidance and immediately asking questions, like dating someone and instantly making requests. We wouldn't do that; we would get to know the relationship. People often expect instant answers, but if you ask a question, it needs to be open-ended, giving your guidance space to answer. If you're looking for an instant answer, you're actually searching your mind, which can only search its data banks and the past. It doesn't hold a higher truth or the path to elevation.

But if you leave it open-ended, have you ever experienced asking the right question, giving it space, and then suddenly, while walking in nature or in the shower, the knowing comes to you? That is your guidance. Your guidance and intuition are like muscles—the more you use them, the more they expand.

When I started developing my gifts, I began with Advanced Holistic Kinesiology. I would look at others with their gifts—some were clairvoyant, others clairaudient—but I felt like I didn't have any gifts. I didn't understand why I felt sick all the time. It was really awful—I just felt really, really sick, heightened, overwhelmed. As I went through this process of elimination, healing myself and doing the work, I remember speaking to a lady once and telling her that I didn't feel like I had any gifts. She responded, "What do you mean? I think you're one of the most intuitive people in this whole program. What you're doing is amazing."

She said, "You feel things intently." I replied, "I know, but I don't have anything else." She explained, "That's called clairsentience. Clearsentience is actually a gift. With your spiritual connection, you need to understand how it works and how it answers you; otherwise, you're missing all of this information." For me, it started with clearsentience, feeling things intensely.

When you start exploring the world of energy, your energy starts to test things. For me, I began playing with energy. I'd be told something, read or learn something, which made my conscious awareness become engaged, and my energetics would always expand it.

I have now expanded my gifts beyond clearsentience into claircognizance, with the strongest being clairaudience, which enables me to hear the truths and stories of my clients at their highest soul aspects.

This is what I hope for you through this book. I hope that some of these ideas unlock pathways, unlock deeper intelligence within you, and unlock the next piece of information for your healing and spiritual expansion journey.

I've had people say that when I talk, they get all tingly. Yes, that's a confirmation or an activation. It resonates and wakes something up inside of you.

Someone once told me about Kundalini energy, and I couldn't even feel these shifts in my body. They described its circular flow like a clock, and I thought, *I didn't know that.* So, I started a process where I would go outside, run my energy, and tune in to each centre in my body along with the Earth. I began to feel things shifting and got really good at this. It was another starting place. As I felt things shift, I could feel when they stopped.

I could feel there was a block, and I would work on releasing it. As I developed further, I started writing. I love writing and channelling. There's a technique called "ghost-writing" where if you clear your mind enough, you can hear higher wisdom come through. It's a process of getting away from the mind. For a long time, my writings stemmed from fear-based programs in my mind. But as I got better at clearing my mind, I dedicated time to myself every day. As I progressed, I started channelling more information and improved, eventually writing and channelling guidance for others.

Then it progressed further, and now I am a medium with clairaudience. I have all the senses, but clairsentience, clairaudience, and claircognizance are predominant. What I'm trying to convey is that you need to know your own connection. If you can feel these shifts within you, you have more power to identify stress, work through things, and release them. Spiritual connection is about getting to know yourself. However, there is also a mixing of the physical with the spiritual.

The physical is created through action. I see many people constantly living in spiritual realms, doing all this manifestation work, and living by the principle of "let's put it in the quantum, and it will manifest." It doesn't work that way. Essentially, yes, but it doesn't. When you put something into the quantum field, you must also remove everything opposing it. That's the healing and manifestation process—they work via the same rules, laws, and principles. But I see people endlessly doing spiritual backing up without taking any action in their lives. You have to take action to cement it into physical form.

People can change their karma through karma. Many have the wrong idea about what it means. Karma is not about doing something good to get something good. It is the energetic mechanism between a choice and its consequence. The more choices I make, the more energetic quality or consequence they have. Many people live by the principle of being loving and giving, but it depends on the quality of the action. For instance, if someone asks me to go to the movies or go out and I don't really want to, but I think, *Oh, that would be a good thing to do,* it's not truly aligned with my genuine desire. That would be a nice thing to do, so I say yes. However, it doesn't affirm me because it's based on obligation, and all I'll get back is more obligation. Be mindful of what you are creating for yourself because the energetic qualities behind your actions are what matter. This is why it's so important to heal those unconscious beliefs. People might spend their whole lives pleasing others.

When I heal EBV, I'm really addressing the underlying root causes of a person's entire life and their stresses. People might have a loving presence, but if it's motivated by lack, disassociation, a need to please, or a desire for everyone to like them due to low self-esteem, love as sacrifice, or other reasons, they end up with more lack. We are all different at the level of our soul, here to experience ourselves as separate beings. The idea that we all should live from our heart space and be interconnected doesn't always work. There are misteachings and generic ideas being rehashed repeatedly. My knowledge now comes from working in the energetics field, not from books. I work with many people who have exceptional gifts.

Don't get me wrong, love and connection in our heart space are beautiful, but that's not everyone's makeup. Some people need to function more from their personal power or wisdom. If they were forced to sit in their heart space, it wouldn't affirm them. I see many spiritual teachings and healers in the marketplace, but it's often just rehashed, regurgitated information. They're saying things but not really saying anything meaningful. Everyone's energetic makeup is completely different.

There is also so much information and many spiritual connections available today. Some people need to be more connected to the Earth, which serves as their platform or highest support and guidance. Multi-dimensional teachings might take them out of alignment with themselves. Different teachings have different multi-dimensional beings or gateways attached to them. If it is not right for you and your energetics, it creates a restriction. This day and age is amazing because there are so many things to learn.

It doesn't mean all the information is right for you. You can take pieces, but you have to make it your own. It's the same as the internet—there are billions, trillions of pieces of information. It doesn't mean it's all correct, and it doesn't mean it's all correct for me. People often say they've been told it was their destiny to suffer. I've had people say their Akashic records indicated that these restrictions were their destiny. Yes, you're playing out these things. Many lifetimes involve restrictions of suffering from illness, and it's playing out in this one, so you can change it. We're our own creators and destroyers. But often, people are afraid of change, afraid to remove things from their lives.

There's a place called the void, the highest level of the throat chakra, which is about change and transitioning through states of consciousness. The mind often sees change as a "death" and wants to hold on because it doesn't have the faith and trust that soul aspects have. It holds onto things and creates more restrictions. Surrendering to the process and trusting the higher path and progression of the soul requires faith in the unseen world. If you create the space, your soul will speak, but the mind has to be quiet.

For a long time, I admit that the spirit scared me a little. At times in my journey, I was in over my head due to my gifts with dark entities. I talk about the superstition model that people run, feeling as though the power is outside of me. It felt like everything was happening to me—all the signs and pathways opening up. I often liken it to following breadcrumbs, expanding one thing after another, healing, and extending my gifts and skills. For me, trust and faith took a long time to develop. I had this fear encased in it as well, trying to make sense of it all. The spiritual doesn't work in a linear fashion like the mind does, so the pieces sometimes feel like they don't fit together. If I tried to work it all out at the level of my mind, it wouldn't come from that place. We're not meant to think about our life; we're meant to feel it.

This is why feelings and emotions are so important. I realised that often I would be asking for a sign, and then the sign wouldn't be good enough, so I'd ask, "Please show me another sign, please show me another sign." This was almost negating the sign. I felt like I was being thrown around by the spiritual. It took me a long time to realise it was always myself, my highest form, calling me home to myself. People often ask me how I knew these things were right. At the time, I didn't know. I would say I just knew what was right and what wasn't, but that's not entirely true. At one point, I didn't know. I just knew what wasn't right, and I kept working on the pieces, releasing, healing, and expanding myself over and over again. The safest connection is the one you facilitate through yourself with time, care, and dedication. I teach people how to tune in to their connection and how to heal and develop themselves.

All the dimensions are interlinked, and when it comes to healing, each holds equal importance. I see many people trying to heal EBV by looking at it one-dimensionally, but you need to link EBV to all dimensions and work with all at the same time.

This is one of my best skills: working across all dimensions at once.

The Earth is the centre (1D), and recalibration needs to occur through this. The Telluric realms (2D) don't answer to the spiritual;

they answer to the Earth. But the Earth is her own sovereign being. The Earth responds to human universal expansion, light frequencies, and elevated consciousness. To regulate the central nervous system, you must do it through the brain. Regulating the brain must be done through the spirit. To create lasting transformation, *soul* transformation is required. People can even be locked out of their connection to the Earth. They can have the polarity points in their body misaligned. We're electromagnetic beings with different points in the body, and they can be out of place. Even though we think we're on the Earth and connecting, we're not.

Lately, I've found that people's thymus cannot update. The thymus is a key structure in multi-dimensional communication and plays a huge role in the immune system. The Earth is shifting a lot, changing her frequency. If we can't shift with her, it creates energetic disruption. It's like we're not grounded or aligned. Minerals, vitamins, and other frequencies are changing, and it's like we're trying to access an outdated matrix that doesn't exist anymore. So, even this connection to the Earth, updating and shifting with her, and shifting with human expansion, helps us absorb life, stay in alignment, and utilise all these frequencies correctly in the body.

I have developed an energetic template for healing EBV. This exists within me, a mixture of research and understanding the virus from information that exists in the world. However, the keys to my knowledge come from expanding this into the spiritual realm.

Having a platform of conscious awareness allowed me to engage with the virus from a physical body level, find the virus in my own body, and create a process to heal it. Over time, working with hundreds of clients, I found the same interlinks and pathways to destruction. But I also found that each person holds unique information—innate intelligence, body, and soul wisdom—the key pieces that allowed this virus to build up in their mind, body, and energetics.

As I worked with this virus in depth, I began to channel more and more higher spiritual information about it, the interlinks to a world in decline, to a person's past, and to dark energy and dark entity interference.

My knowledge does not come from books; it comes from working directly with the virus and the energetics that surround it. The template to heal EBV exists within me, in my spiritual and energetic frameworks. The gifts I have enhanced within myself enable me to realise that it is possible to bring the virus back into balance within the human energy field. With all these gifts to heal the virus—mind, body, and soul—I also have the ability to use a very powerful multi-dimensional frequency to bring the virus into submission, to recode the energetics of the virus to stop it from reactivating.

## Chapter Summary

In this chapter, I have explored the spiritual and energetic dimensions of healing from EBV. I discussed how our physical body is the gateway to our spiritual and soul aspects and how EBV can create blocks to these higher connections. I explained the concept of the "dark night of the soul" and how it relates to the healing journey. I also elucidated the different dimensions of existence and the importance of understanding energy and vibrational frequencies in the healing process. Sharing my own experiences with developing my intuitive gifts and the role of the liver in spiritual reconnection, I emphasised the importance of reconnecting with our spiritual guidance and innate intelligence to facilitate true healing and transformation.

**Channelled Message** (divine guidance that speaks poetically, awakening a deep, heightened sense of knowing and truth within.)

*We live in a world of instant triggers and associations*
*At times watching and waiting for an intervention*
*Secret knowledge bases destined to secure elevation, designed to bring unity to any unruly structure or misalignment*
*Balance is key*
*Balance is unseen*
*Balance is restored, always softly spoken*
*The unmanifest of the divine templates reorders physicality, reorders malnourishment within the human psyche*
*Always*
*Mind over matter creates disruption but the soul creates so much more*
*Natural alliances to love reconnection and to the correct wisdom*
*Wisdom so potent it is the secret to restoring humanities long lost directive*
*The soul and its unspoken rulings*
*The soul will always secure freedoms of time and space*
*Freedoms in the form of unlocking one's true and only path progression forward.*

## CHAPTER 6

# Entities

As I mentioned, I didn't even realise that I was a spiritual being. So, the world of energy came to me as a big surprise. My starting foundation was Advanced Holistic Kinesiology, and I feel really blessed to have this as my starting place. Australia and New Zealand are the most advanced in the world for this amazing therapy. The specific diploma I studied was world-class. The head instructor, who was also the course content creator, is exceptional, and his information was so in-depth and profound.

As I started learning and began my intense journey into self and healing, it was like opening Pandora's box. Although my foundations came from this starting point, the making of me came from navigating the darkness. It's almost like I had these gifts that can't be learned from a book or a teacher. I had soul gifts in my energetic makeup, but I had no idea as most of my life I was so shut down.

For a long time, I didn't understand this and didn't have a handle on it. I was like a new wizard wielding magic that I had no idea how to use. I didn't know what these gifts meant or how dark things could actually get for me.

The head trainer at the time, who had around 30 years of experience in healing and teaching, said at the start of my journey how strange it was that I had so many entities attached to me. He only knew 1%, not even that. He didn't know about my journey or the levels of entity interference that I was dealing with.

I was seeing another healer at the time. She was qualified in the same modality I was currently training in but had also started to include many other types of energetic healings, as well as entity release techniques. She was also shocked and said to me that with the number of dark entities and the amount of dark energy I had, anyone else would be dead.

As I started to progress, I had so much to shift and clear, always linked to dark entity interference. The dark energy and dark entities made me feel constantly sick.

At that point in time, my main gift was clearsentience, although I didn't know or understand this. I simply knew that I felt sick a lot, and when there was a dark presence attached, it would heighten this feeling within me. It was really scary, and I felt out of control for a long time, which had negative consequences for me trying to live a normal life as a wife and mother of three children.

So, I pretty much felt sick all the time. It was really awful not understanding what was happening, what was going on, or how to work with these energies. But the healer I was working privately with at the time thought she was doing me a favour by giving me more energetic information. She gave me instructions for a whole new modality called Holographic Kinetics, which deals with multi-dimensional entities and offers a technique for releasing them.

This in itself is dangerous, as when you learn something, your energy will test it. With any modality, there is much more to consider. To learn and use any new healing modality you need to energetically update to be able to use it correctly and safely.

There's a whole process to learning Holographic Kinetics. It teaches you how to release entities, but if they don't comply, you lock them away into another dimension. So I had all this new information. As I said, your energy will always test something. I didn't realise how powerful my energy was or what could happen. This is the point where it got so far out of hand for me; it was terrifying in the end. If I had known what I was getting into, I would have said no.

At one point, I was in so deep, so over my head, and my mantra was, "When you are going through hell, don't stop." Dark night of the soul—I couldn't even tell you how many I've had or how long I stayed in them. It was frightening.

The founder and head trainer of the kinesiology class I was taking later told me he does not teach anyone entity release or working with entities until nearly the end of the course because you are not ready for it. Your energy could not handle those things, and you would get in over your head. You have to have a sovereign presence. Sovereignty is what we're all trying to achieve. Sovereignty is our right to enact our own destiny without interference. But again, there's a process to reclaim this in a person, and it's through healing and extending someone's soul vibration rate.

My journey was really unmanageable. It's like I opened up to a world that I couldn't control, and it was so dark and so scary. The stories are endless. One day, I'm going to write a book just about entities—some of the stories are unbelievable. I ended up with PTSD from my healing journey. If I wasn't already broken, this was a new level of breaking.

I didn't have many people who could help me because what I was dealing with was either unheard of or there was no one that could help me at these levels. I liken my journey to Hansel and Gretel, just trying to work through one piece at a time. There's a very fine line between sanity and insanity when it comes to the spiritual, unlocking, and developing intuition and spiritual gifts.

I help many people now who end up in situations like I was. In fact, all the things I can do in healing are because I have done them all for myself. I have walked the path, and I can only do the work at these levels because this is my story. This is my journey. I hold the template for all the unique healings I can do, like EBV and soul healing/transformation work, because I've done it all for myself first.

This is so important for healers—they must have healed themselves first and have the energetic template within them to create this for another.

Through the darkness, I did get help. In the last chapter, I spoke about guidance. At one point in my journey, I read a book that discussed vibration and frequency. It was a whole modality using frequency. As I was reading it, my body started tingling, activating things within myself. Not long after that, I was visited by multi-dimensional beings who gave me access to vibrations not found on Earth, allowing me to develop extra healing abilities. I've had so many other experiences like this, which all have interplays with the multi-dimensional healing I do.

Many of the vibrations I use are from dimensions beyond what people's energetics can access. I have tethered some of these to vibrations in the fifth dimension (5D) so I can teach anybody who wants to heal themselves how to access and channel them... It's like a bridge for others to access what I can. Just as I hold the template in my energetics for healing EBV, I also hold the template for many other healings and vibrations that I continually offer to my clients for healing themselves or for use in their healing practices with their own clients.

The light guided and supported me, along with the channelled learnings and teachings. Most of what I do in my healing techniques now is not learned from others. They come directly from my own connection, working with extremely powerful multi-dimensional beings who have helped me elevate myself, my knowledge, and my gifts to hold these high multi-dimensional frequencies in the form of new knowledge, lessons, and learnings about what is possible in healing.

So, amidst the darkness, there was some beautiful elevation. My gifts to reclaim myself came through the dark, and it was a progression. The things I know about entities are from firsthand experiences and from working with higher and higher levels of energy.

Years ago, I was asked if I would do possession work. Possession is when an entity is actually in a person's physical body. It looks like the stuff out of horror movies.

For quite a while, I declined this because I knew my energetics would not survive it. I've had to attune myself for years because the way I heal people is through energetic surrogacy, where I bring a person's energy into my body. I bring all of their energetic information into my energetic systems, into my body, and then I am able to release and command the energy and entities; some people have thousands, even millions of attachments, and without having someone who can command dark energy and entities at the highest level they will always have restrictions from accessing their highest souls path.

One thing that is very true is the dark tries to derail the light. Most clients I have worked with that have had severe entity interference is because they have untapped gifts and an important soul's purpose that needs to be unlocked in this lifetime.

I get asked a lot if what I do is dangerous. The answer is yes! I see many people, even other healers, accessing energies and activating realms they either don't have permission to access or don't have the gifts to protect themselves and their clients from.

I think I didn't realise how dangerous it was—how much I was putting not just my energy but my body at risk. I spent years working with clients, facing higher restrictions and new levels of entity interference. After each session, I always had to say, "There were no negative side effects for me," but often, there were. This used to be commonplace for me because if a client had a health issue or interference that resonated with my energy, I would have to spend hours, even days, working on my own energy to heal the resonance in myself. This is why my healing journey, especially when it came to entity interference, was relentless. If you think the complexities we deal with in our physical bodies are vast, they are nothing compared to the infinite levels of multi-dimensional and spiritual realms.

At one point, my husband asked me why I was working this way, using my body as a tool and often as a sacrifice. This was when I would have restrictions, entities, and many other things that would create endless issues for me. It was affecting my life and relationships as I had to pull away and work on myself all the time. I'm so grateful my husband supported me through this journey and believed in me even when he was scared and worried for my life and sanity.

Over time, my presence and abilities grew stronger and stronger. Now, I can work at the highest levels possible and would never shy away from any entity issue, for I am beyond that. I've had to work through many blocks and restrictions heightened by dark entities. What you need to know about entities is that they need a loophole or an attachment mechanism, and I had to heal or close all of mine. This is why understanding the interplay between dark entities, dark energy, and EBV is so important. EBV creates so many restrictions on all dimensions of our being, so the loopholes and attachment mechanisms are vast for entities and dark energy to access. But please note, no two clients are the same when it comes to entity interference; we all have our own unique blueprint, unique soul, and unique life stories. So it's not just one entity. EBV is not an entity; it creates the loopholes and attachment mechanisms for multiple entity interferences, which add the highest layer of restriction on a person's energetics. This is why millions of people suffer from health issues like EBV.

I will explain the types of entities later in this chapter.

Mastering entity interference has definitely been a progression. It's taken me years to attune my energetics to work at these levels. Now, I work at the highest levels of dark entities, which means I do the highest levels of spiritual healing and light work possible.

A lot of people think there is only one level of light. There is not. Many have naive views that light and dark fight each other and that light always wins.

That's not the case at all. If somebody is wielding a level of light but there is an entity at a higher dark level, that darkness has more power than the light and will win. When it comes to entity work, you have to have something called governance. You have to be at a higher state of being, at a higher level of power, to command something. Otherwise, you cannot. People get into a lot of trouble. I hear lots of healers saying, "Just show them the light." I'll explain the different types of entities in a minute. They don't belong in the light. Maybe a few might go with that, but they would be low-level entities. It's a naive view. If you're viewing the spiritual as only light, you're missing half of the equation.

I work with many gifted people who have extra abilities in the form of an "Oversoul." An Oversoul is a multi-dimensional being that co-creates with humanity. It gives them additional abilities and manifestations, among a number of other gifts.

Sometimes, people sell courses and talk about manifestation. They teach you the principles and talk about multimillion-dollar frequencies and other things. Some of these people have exceptional gifts and abilities because they have a multi-dimensional presence attached to them that helps them. It's not just commonplace. So again, there's all this misinformation in the market. People don't really understand how some of these things truly work. For me to be able to work with people who have exceptional gifts, such as those with Oversouls and unique energetics, I have to be able to contain and hold both these energetics and the physical person's energetics.

This is why choosing a healer is so important—one who has healed themselves and done the work and continues to do the work. They need to be expanded in their own soul vibration rate; all of these factors play a significant role. If they're not at the level to see high restrictions, like high dark entity interference, it's not even on their radar—they can't see it, so they can't advise or help you at the highest levels.

As we progress in our journey and become more energetically attuned, this can be a downfall for some people. When I talked before about the spiritual being a wonderful place, people get wooed by it, get all excited, and start doing more and more spiritual healing work. They start setting more and more intentions. We create our reality through intentions, right?

That's the starting place. But when we set more and more intentions, we attract something called white and blue lights. We are given extra guidance that supports us. Blue lights are a form of multi-dimensional beings that uphold and amplify our intentions in the quantum field. They are not as extreme as an Oversoul—that's a different thing altogether. Sometimes, I see people doing a lot of spiritual work but actually disempowering themselves because they over-create. They've got this amplification on manifestation because they've done so much of it. They're working with those principles, but they have other restrictions, and it actually amplifies more quickly for them.

This is the path I went down. I started creating everything from negative intent. My life got very, very out of control very, very quickly. It's like I created more and more programs and restrictions on top of my healing journey. Manifestations occurred at an unprecedented rate, with terrible misalignments, and my energetics were creating all of it.

At one point, I was working with a very experienced, well-known marketing person. Their strategy for brand positioning and "putting yourself out in the world" was to state that you were the best in the world at something.

This was a few years ago, and at that point in time, I said, "I can't do this. I cannot claim I'm the best in the world if I'm not." I would never say that. I would never do that. I understand the repercussions from an entity interference perspective. It would not be worth my life to claim that I was the best in the world in the realms of dark entities because those highest dark entities would make my life a living hell.

You do not want to draw attention to yourself if you do not have the skills to back it up.

This has been my journey. Now, I can say hand on heart that I am one of the best in the world at entity removal and work at the highest levels of dark energy and dark entity interference without compromise!

Now, I would like to explain to you that there are different types of entities that play by very different sets of rules. They include demonic realms and multi-dimensional interference.

## Demonic Realms

Demonic realms include entities like demons. They feed off suffering and answer to the devil. Yes, he does exist—the Prince of Darkness. It's almost like they are assigned by him.

They heighten restrictions that are already there, feeding off suffering, shame, guilt, and all the low frequencies in a person's energetics. They create more and more disconnection and can intensify physical blocks and restrictions, interfere with your mind and thought processes, and heighten feelings and emotions.

There are different roles for different entities. Over the years, I've learned many techniques. I was often asked if I would teach someone what I knew, and I always said I would never do that. I would never put anyone in the situation I've been in because I would not want them to go through what I had to. I don't know how many people could have handled it without losing their minds—or worse, their lives.

I had a healer come to me who thought she was dealing with an entity issue within a property she worked in. However, it was a personal issue. She was working in a healing space, which is rife with entity interference due to people releasing entities during their healing sessions. If the healer doesn't have the skills or gifts to transcend the entities, they will hang around the space, looking for the next person to attach to.

The entities in this space were causing many issues for her, not just in her energetics but also physically hurting her, clawing at her feet, and creating endless issues in her energy and health.

I told her she had issues with entities and that she needed to heal and clear her energetic boundaries. She needed to clear the programs she was running.

I often find that the healers who have the most dark entities and dark entity interference are usually the ones who have the ability to work with entities but haven't developed the skills. If they're overlooking this very thing and not working with dark entities and dark energies, then they are not stepping into their full power. This will always cause a huge problem in all areas of life. This refers back to the number of healers and lightworkers who only focus on the light.

Entities can see all your unclaimed gifts and spiritual matrices. This is what they're looking for. They like to tap into lightworkers or healers. I always said I wouldn't teach entity removal, but when this person came to me, I was told to create a new modality to teach the world how to engage and command entities in a safe way with no backlash or repercussions. When I worked with the technique of

Holographic Kinetics, there was a method where you would lock something away in a different dimension. You better hope it doesn't get back out—believe me, it can. All these things can amplify, and if you can't see all the details, it's really, really frightening. You need the right tools to clear entities. For demonic realms, the command and release sends them back to the devil.

## Multidimensional Interference

Then, there are multi-dimensional entities and interference. Multi-dimensional entities make demonic entities look like a walk in the park. When I talked about the dimensions earlier, you would read in books that there are ten dimensions. Yes, regarding physicality and humanness, there are ten dimensions we recognise. But the universe is different; there are hundreds of dimensions. At one point, I didn't understand this or know it.

As my journey progressed, starting from my healing journey and learning Advanced Holistic Kinesiology, entity interference was my biggest restriction. That's why it's been the biggest area of my growth and expansion, because I have to work at the highest multi-universal (multi-dimensional) levels to address multi-dimensional interference.

I could tell you hundreds of stories about everything new I learned and everything I had to heal for myself and my clients—literally everything went hand in hand with entities, including Epstein-Barr virus.

Because of my skills and gifts with multi-dimensional entities, I do a lot of Earth grid interference work as well as multiverse engagement. Most healers and lightworkers would know this level as working with the Galactic Federation of Light.

What you need to understand about multi-dimensional beings is that they cut into someone's connection at their tenth-dimensional aspect, posing a huge problem. They create significant misalignment and disconnection in someone's spiritual frameworks and connection. They feed off energetics; we are like an energy source to them. Often, I see these entities compromise a healer, and then, for every person the healer engages with, the multi-dimensional beings gain access to their energetics as well.

It's like syphoning a person's energy and life force energetics, but more importantly, they claim people's unclaimed spiritual potential.

These are the types of entities that can literally derail a person's life, causing huge health declines, mental health issues, and manipulating thought patterns. This creates massive misalignment with a person's manifestation abilities and alignment to their soul's purpose and path progression.

If a healer doesn't have the ability to work at these levels or with these types of energies, they can't even see them, and the healing session will often be at a level lower than the restriction. This means you'll be in an endless search and healing practice without addressing the highest issue.

There's a whole different command with multi-dimensional beings. Power respects power. If you're not at a level of command, it can't be done. I've heard stories of people fighting with entities for hours, and they tell it like they're wearing a badge of honour about how they can do this entity work. If you have to fight with an entity for hours, you do not have governance over it. You cannot command it. Maybe you'll fight long enough that it leaves, but it will come back. Fighting with entities is not commanding them.

Governance and commanding in that way keep someone safe. I only know these things because it took me a very long time to work at these levels. Entities don't just do these things to us— as mentioned, they need an attachment mechanism or a loophole to create a restriction for someone. Remember, the universe doesn't judge us; it just reads our energetic matrix and the energetic rules we are running.

Entities can see all of our spiritual matrices. They can see all our holes. If there's a likeness, they can attach to it, especially if a healer or another, for that matter, is running programs that take on other people's energetics and entities.

There are so many factors. When someone has an entity issue, I often hear people say, "I need to protect myself." Well, if you're trying to protect yourself, it's coming from fear. This creates more restrictions, more fear, and more entity interference. It's about stepping into power, into sovereignty, and healing the reason why the entity was there or could connect with you in the first place.

When it comes to commanding entities, you often have to hear the full reason for the attachment and heal this area of a person's life before the entity can be removed.

So, how do Epstein-Barr virus and entities fit together?

As mentioned in previous pages, all blocks and restrictions go hand in hand with dark energy and dark entities. It's simply the way it works. I've also spoken many times about EBV feeding off our stress responses, creating the pathway for it to increase. In order to heal, you have to find the key pieces in someone's life. You have to find their key triggers for stress or their misalignments and heal those things at the same time. Not everyone's main issue will be entities.

Some people I see have extreme entity interference, which is the sole reason for EBV building up. For some people who come to me to heal EBV, I have to find their key pieces, and for some, it is all about entity interference. It is this interference that has stifled their energetic systems. Healers often have the highest levels of entity interference because they work in those realms doing spiritual work. By opening yourself up to more entity interference, the dark tries to derail the light. This is why my journey has been so hard and why I now have the most powerful gifts for commanding entities—because I had to rise above all of them.

Another major attachment mechanism is something called "mistaken identity." Mistaken identity occurs when a person thinks they are engaging and speaking directly with the light. Remember, I have said time and time again that the spiritual is not all love and light.

People will often do anything and even give up their own sovereignty in the promise of connection. This looks like someone thinking they are talking to a light being when, often, dark beings will be posing as the light. They'll pose as angels or light beings. Many people get so excited about the spiritual that they talk to various beings without knowing who or what they are communicating with, or they channel energy without understanding what is behind it. Entities create a lot of trickery and are very deceitful. I would not recommend just chatting away to them. I've seen whole spiritual teachings where someone claims they are channelling John the Beloved, and I've had to do work for several people who came out of it, and it was not John the Beloved but entities masking as him.

Mistaken identity is an attachment mechanism right there. It's almost like you're saying yes because you're not energetically discerning.

One good question is, "Are you of positive intent?" If you ask an entity directly, they have to answer with yes or no. But people get excited. I see so many people these days doing spiritual activation healings or attuning people to higher frequencies without knowing what they are activating.

They don't even know what they're activating or opening up. I have seen the spiritual make people very, very sick. I have seen people go to healers and become extremely unwell afterwards, not knowing what was wrong with them. Unfortunately, they had just had a session with a compromised healer.

The number of compromised healers is greater than most people think. Many healers with heightened multi-dimensional interference will compromise the people they come in contact with. Also, a lot of compromised healers get so worn down that they stop doing healing work and following their highest path.

Not everybody's main issue is entity interference; however, it's important to understand that entities go hand in hand with all blocks and restrictions. This can lead to huge health declines, illness, and disease, just like EBV.

I've seen many Reiki attunements go horribly wrong for people. Not all Reiki practitioners are equal; it depends on who they were taught by and what frequencies they are channelling. There isn't just one level of light; there are many. You're channelling some form of it, but it might not be what you think you're channelling. Sometimes, the frequency is full of entity interference and attachments.

We need to create energetic boundaries. Maybe we're taking too much on—such as an empath, taking on other people's pain. I'm sorry, you're not just taking their pain; there are lots of other things that people can't see. Over time, those things will stifle energetics and wear a person down. And I'm sorry to tell you, but there is actually more entity transference in spiritual circles than anywhere else. You'll understand that places and things like bars, alcohol, drugs, porn etc, all hold low levels of consciousness that attract a lot of entity interference, but it is also the same in many spiritual healing circles.

When people do group healing, they release their trauma, and with it, they release their dark entities. Unless a facilitator releases, clears and works directly with the entities, they simply hang around and reattach somewhere else. It took me a long time to work this out. I've seen people go to healing sessions and release three issues, but they pick up another eight. Often, people wonder why they're not making any headway in their healing; this can be a large contributing factor, constantly picking up more and more entity interference.

I hear this all the time: people in spiritual circles constantly dealing with physical attacks; this is the same thing. At one point in my journey, I didn't understand how this worked; I just knew that I was constantly having to deal with attack after attack. My journey through constant entity interference at the highest of levels created C-PTSD in itself, making the journey unbearable at times. I was often so, so unwell. I couldn't work it out. It was horrible and scary.

I came out of three years of study and experienced an amazing transformation, but wow, was it hard. My husband booked me a retreat because he could see that I was at my breaking point. I went away to this retreat where they did sound healing. There was a guy there with a gong. I didn't know at the time that gongs were historically used to cast out demons.

In this room, there were about 30 people. After the healing, I couldn't even move. I was so sick; I didn't understand what had happened. I thought maybe I was just integrating, but I couldn't even eat with people. I had to go to bed. It was horrible. I had to remove thousands and thousands of entities from me. Bearing in mind my energetic system, I didn't realise at the time that I was designed to work with entities. My energetic structures are very different; it was like moths to a flame. So, I would have picked up everything in the room. They all would have come to me.

When I went home from that retreat, I was sick. It took me ages to unwind all of the restrictions and entity attachments that I had picked up. I didn't understand what was going on at the time. I remember reaching out to the person who led the retreat, and he just said, "Oh, you probably started an activation but didn't finish it." At the same retreat, there was someone convulsing on the floor who couldn't get up. I now see many stories like this—spiritual healing circles creating huge entity interference for a person. They know something is wrong at the time, but it's sold to them as an awakening or an activation, and they just have more layers to work through.

Even though I would like to tell people not to go to group healing sessions, as healing is a very private thing, I do not, as I feel for some, the connection, working on themselves, doing the healing work, and experiencing the divine holds so much value and many lessons. For this reason, I have created a solution: a programmed crystal that transcends entities, specially designed for use in group healing sessions and for lightworkers and healers who do not have the skills to work directly with entities. It safeguards their energetic bodies, disallowing new entity interference to occur. One of my clients attended a festival where the crystal had transcended 834 entities within two hours. Environments with dense energies and overstimulation become bearable when wearing this programmed crystal.

I helped a man recently who was deeply unwell. He originally wanted to speak to me about EBV, although when he told me his story, I felt profoundly sorry for him as his main issue was entity interference from an incident 30 years earlier. The entity was so powerful it had created so much mental and physical health decline over decades. When he was younger, he had travelled to many places overseas looking for spiritual lessons and enlightenment. He visited a Buddhist monk retreat—somewhere amazing for reconnection and spiritual growth. He had set the intention that he wanted to feel the most powerful energy that was there. He had this awakening where his body was convulsing. After that, it was like this energy was moving through him, and he didn't know what to do. It was awful. He was really unwell and went on a search for the next person to help him, moving from place to place. He went to another Kundalini place, and they sold it to him as a Kundalini awakening.

He got sicker and sicker as he felt this energy in his body; he used to have to get up in the middle of the night and discharge the uncontrollable energetics into the Earth. Over time, his condition worsened, and his body stopped working properly. He was always convulsing and continued to lose control over his body and health.

He came to me as a last resort, bearing in mind this was 30 years later. I told him he had entity interference from the time he set the intention to receive the most powerful, intense energy. Unfortunately, he had brought in the most intense dark entity interference into his physical body (entity interference at the level of a person's physical body is classed as possession), and it had completely ruined his life.

I did the work for him and released his entity issue. However, you need to understand that an entity of this magnitude, over the course of 30 years, had created such energetic disruptions that it then led to physical decline and serious health issues.

The physical body takes time to heal, so after removing the entities, you need to continue to heal and repair the damage caused on all levels of your being—mind, body, energy, and soul.

That's an extreme story.

I had another woman come to visit me. I don't normally see people in person; I usually do all my work through energetic surrogacy. However, she lived near me and was a healer. She told me she thought her connection had been compromised. She couldn't hear anything for herself. A lot of healers tell me they can't even tune in to their own connection properly, but when they work for other people, it's clear, and they can offer healing to their clients. This is a huge problem because you should be able to tune into your connection for yourself.

I asked her how she was healing and what she was doing. She dealt with entities. I asked, "How do you clear entities? What are you doing?"

She replied, "Oh, I breathe them into my lungs and blow them out into a bowl of water."

I asked, "Who taught you that?"

She said it was a shaman technique. So I told her, "That's a very, very unsafe technique. How do you know you're getting rid of them all?"

She sounded like she was about to cry and said, "I don't."

So I invited her to see me.

When she turned up at my house, my little Cavoodle dog, who is so placid and never barks, started going crazy. She started barking at her and wouldn't go near her. I ignored it and said to her, "Sit down." I could see that she had multiple entities in her physical lung space.

As soon as I released all of the entities and interference that were attached to her, my little dog jumped up on her knee and started licking her face. She started crying and said, "I knew why your dog was barking."

I then showed her other techniques, such as vibrations that would release entities through her hands. I told her never to do that technique again because when I did the work for her, I heard entities laughing—laughing at the stupidity and knowing they wouldn't go into a bowl of water.

I see people using sage, clearing properties, and burying crystals in the Earth. Crystals are not going to release a high multi-dimensional entity. They might not even release a demonic presence, perhaps just fractured energies.

There are many different types of energies.

So when a healer says to simply show an entity the light, maybe if it was an earthbound soul that wasn't compromised, this might work. But there are many, many types of entities. I've seen houses ruin people's lives.

I do a lot of property clearing for clients and real estate agents who come to me for properties that aren't selling.

I had a client in Melbourne with a multimillion-dollar house that was beautiful, but they couldn't sell it. Every time they tried to sell it, all these things would go wrong.

The agent hired me to clear this beautiful old mansion that dated back to a shipping tycoon as the original owner. This man thought his wife was having an affair, lost his mind, and eventually killed his wife and himself in the house.

Everybody who owned the house afterwards had nothing but demise and problems, but the current owner thought the property was so amazing and had these beautiful architraves that he believed if he restored the property and loved it, things would change.

It had been seven years, and his wife's health had declined over this time. She had gotten very sick. There was even a room in the house that they wouldn't go into—everybody knew not to go into it. They could feel it, and it was really awful energy. He said the house had ruined his life. I said, "What a shame." I asked if he could stay if I cleared it for him because he had put so much love into it.

He said, "No, it's done too much damage to our health and life."

I said, "What a shame because everything can be changed if you know how to do it and work with energy." I cleared the property, helping move the energy and entities on. Within two weeks, the property sold after a year on the market.

When I hear people's life stories and ask them about Epstein-Barr Virus (EBV), I often guide them to pinpoint the moment when their health began to decline. By asking the right questions and revisiting significant events from their past, we usually identify key moments in time. For some, it's a single pivotal event, while for others, it's a series of compounding experiences that lead to complete disconnection from their true self and a severe decline in health.

I've worked with many healers who assist clients with entity removal and interference, but I've found that some become compromised. Either they lack the ability to clear their own attachments, or the entities they're dealing with are at such a high level that they can't perceive or remove them. I also work with people who are constantly exposed to trauma and suffering in environments like mental hospitals, prisons, crematoriums, and end-of-life care.

One person who stands out to me is a compassionate end-of-life veterinarian. Her job involved not only caring for pets but also supporting their grieving owners. Over time, her empathetic nature became overwhelmed as she absorbed others' grief, and she became entangled in the darker energies surrounding death and trauma. This wasn't just emotional strain or unprocessed trauma—it was constant interaction with entities that fed on the heavy energies in her environment. She described feeling haunted by thoughts of death and unable to find peace. Her health and mind deteriorated to the point where she was experiencing a constant dark night of the soul. When I tested her for EBV, her levels were over 90%—one of the highest I had ever seen.

In many cases, mental health struggles can result from an overstressed brain, but they can also involve significant entity interference. Removing these dark energies was the first step toward helping this beautiful soul regain her sovereignty and restore her mental and physical health.

I've heard other stories of repeated freak accidents, like falling down stairs and feeling as though they were pushed, manifestations going horribly wrong, healing work being sabotaged, and darkness being amplified endlessly. My heart breaks for these people because I know firsthand what it feels like to be in that place. Often, these energies cause a slow decline, and by the time someone realises they've been compromised, it's been years—sometimes even decades—in the making.

This is why the spiritual becomes endless for people—often, it is because they're just picking up more and more entity interference.

I've spoken about mistaken identity. I see people talking about channelling hundreds and thousands of beings.

How are you channelling? What's the being?

You have to be aware of all the energetics and information, or you open yourself up to misaligned misinformation and attachment mechanisms.

I've seen whole modalities that claim to be of the light. They speak of the higher mind, the mind that connects to the source, as the insane mind.

They also claim there is only one entity of the insane mind that needs to be removed, and they release this entity through abbreviations and acronyms. The person reciting these commands doesn't even understand what they are saying or instructing, and it's actually implanting more entities at the level of a person's mind. This makes me sick, and I have seen it change people's personalities, disconnect them from the source, and create the very insanity they believed they were clearing.

I know this firsthand because I've tried some of these modalities and come away with more restrictions and entity interference. At one stage of my journey, when personal vibrational healing devices came onto the market, I was asked if I would try this vibrational device and use it for my clients.

I was told by my guidance to try this device as there was a message for me, and I can't comment or recommend anything if I haven't used it and brought it into my energetics.

So I went along, and they asked for my date of birth and name to put into this device. I said, "I'm sorry, I won't give you that information." I asked, "Who gets it? Where does it go?"

Giving someone that information grants access to your spiritual frameworks and spiritual matrixes. I would never do that.

Who's it linking to? What energetics are behind it? What multidimensional beings are behind that device? Because there's always a connection to spiritual realms.

The person couldn't answer any of these questions, so I said, "I can't give you that information. I'm sorry. I'm not comfortable with that." But I asked if I could still try the device. I tried it, and my body liked it. I could tell my body really liked it. It did offer a level of healing, but when I went home, I had so many misalignments at a spiritual level that I had to go through a process of releasing them all. Then, I was directed to create new vibrational frequencies that people could use in healing without compromise and restriction to their spiritual frameworks.

I was told I would create five new vibrational frequencies. That would bring healing and restoration to the physical as well as spiritual healing and expansion. Many of the vibrations I work with have taken me years and years to attune my energetics and my body to. Other people wouldn't be able to hold the energetics because they don't have the platform in their physical body. Even to do the work I do, I've had to change my physical structures over and over again to elevate and hold these powerful frequencies.

So I created a program with five different vibrational frequencies that people can access—ones you've felt at some point in your life—but I've tethered them to a higher vibrational frequency. So when you access one vibration, you're getting access to another one that offers much more healing and support in all different areas, even entity release.

Another huge restriction I see that holds a lot of entity interference is when someone has been in an abusive and dysfunctional relationship, often referred to as a narcissistic relationship. People may have done a lot of healing work over the years on these relationships from a personal aspect. But I always say when you upset someone, you don't worry about the person; you worry about what's attached to them. You worry about the multi-dimensional presence and the dysfunctional energy and attachments responsible for their abusive behaviour.

This is what you have to heal and clear—the interlink to the high entity interference. I would have to break many high connections that almost enslave people and create endless recycling of pain and trauma from their past. It's like they can never step out of the dysfunction of the relationship until this multidimensional interference is cleared. So again, everybody's stresses are different.

I've seen things like this: I had a client who came to me for a property clearing. She thought her property was cursed because she'd had nothing but bad luck in her health and her life. She was a transformational coach who did all this healing work for others and had done endless amounts of healing work on herself. When I did the work for her, I knew I had to do it for free. I said, "I can't charge you for it, and I don't know why until I do the work."

I realised why. Her father had bought a property years ago in Australia, which was sacred Aboriginal land. Her name was on the title. He brought the property to develop it and was told not to move the large rocks on the land because they were sacred and that moving them would bring bad luck. He didn't listen and moved them anyway so he could develop the property for greed and money. This is why I couldn't charge for the clearing, as it could not hold the same energetics, doing something for monetary gain. She told me the story that her father's whole life had disintegrated. He lost everything—his health, his wealth—everything went from bad to worse. She was tied into it, and her father's actions affected her, as she was having similar bad luck.

When I did the work, I realised there was something called a "bloodline curse."

She had done endless work to heal herself and free up what was causing her so much misfortune, but the bloodline curse existed at a higher spiritual level, in a different matrix. These higher dimensional levels exist. She was forever trying to piece back her life by working on Akashic records, unconscious beliefs, and a lot of mental and emotional work. But there was an overarching program or intent that had been placed. It was in a matrix that people would never be able to access; only highly powerful beings have access to it.

I had to release that overarching curse because while it ran in her life, it didn't matter how much healing work she did; it was the overarching program that superseded everything. This is why I'm saying the spiritual can be endless unless you're getting the right pieces. It is about finding the right pieces that are causing the stress, blocks, and restrictions in a person's energetics, as EBV feeds off stress. Identifying the highest cause of the stress that Epstein-Barr virus feeds off is the key to creating lasting healing.

**Ask the question:** What are these key triggers? What are the key pieces, events and triggers that have equated to your stress build-up?

Often, people work with many layers of stress, but there's a key piece that sits really deep. If you can prompt that and look at it, you make more headway in your healing because everything else is an offshoot of the web of sub-creation from this one point in time. You've got to find the key pieces. When dealing with a narcissistic or dysfunctional relationship, when I clear that multi-dimensional presence, it almost sets that person free.

It's like unlocking them. They're suddenly free to have their own sovereignty and enact their own destiny without interference. Some of these things can create such huge interference that they can literally block someone from their own path. I've seen people after Ayahuasca journeys. (Plant medicine)

Ayahuasca is a whole different realm; it's not even a light realm. It's the realm of truth and lies. Dark entities put on a show, offering information. Then people get drawn into the spiritual, thinking everything shown to them during their journey really exists.

It's almost like the movie *The Greatest Showman*. I've seen people open vortexes in their minds, and if I hadn't helped them, they would have gone crazy. I've had a client who died because she didn't come to me for six months after a journey. The amount of entity interference was astounding. She had been completely cut off from the source and got sicker and sicker—it was terrible. She said when she turned up, the guy (shaman) seemed different. She had done work with him before, and he had cancelled this journey at one point because he couldn't handle the energetics. Then, he started charging people thousands of dollars for his Ayahuasca journeys. It makes me feel really angry because so many people now are leading awakening ceremonies without the skills or understanding of the realm they're dealing with. As I said, It's called the realm of truth and lies. People go expecting to see God, but God does not exist there. There's a payment for travelling to that realm, and you better hope the shaman knows how to reclaim what is lost because gifts will be taken in the background. I've seen people think they've had an amazing journey and experience, but they're not aware they've lost part of their path progression or soul gifts. There's more to it than meets the eye.

Your connection is sacred, and there's a way to develop it safely.

There's a way to release your restrictions, which are there for a reason. Even people taking others on journeys—it's actually your consciousness that keeps you safe. When you split from your consciousness, it's extremely dangerous. The intention with plant medicine has changed. It was meant to be a sacred, tribal thing, not for everyone. People seek big spiritual experiences and expanded consciousness, which seem amazing because it's the unseen world. But it's not. You're giving away pieces of your soul gifts and unclaimed potential.

We live in an instant gratification world where people look for shortcuts and quick fixes, applying the same expectations to their spiritual connection. Your spiritual connection is sacred and takes time, discipline, and dedication to enhance. True and lasting transformation should always be the goal.

I have done endless healing within myself, and the darkness always paves the way for the light.

Most people think God and the universe are the same energy, using the terms interchangeably. I thought the same until I had this experience.

This was a pivotal point in my journey. Speaking with God and being in direct communion paved the way for me to receive a reprieve from the devil. I was told, *"Dark energy and dark entities will no longer be allowed to fraternise with you."* At this point, everything changed. I could go places without being constantly bombarded by dark forces.

As you will see, God is for humanity. The universe is very different; it does not judge us. It simply mirrors back our energetics to us. This is key when it comes to manifestation, working with universal rules, laws, and principles.

Multi-dimensional presence and multi-dimensional interference are entirely different. They have no place with God. God doesn't command them, as they are universal and exist in a different dimensional field. This is why there are separate rules for different realms when it comes to entity commands.

I would love to share my message from God with you as it is one of my most cherished channelled messages, and I have permission to share it with you here:

*Today marks a very special day.*
*You are ready to hear what it is that I do.*
*At the beginning of time, I was given grace over mankind, the role of guide, protector, helper—the list goes on.*
*As you know, is struggling to know themselves in physicality.*

*The mind, the ego—many names, interfere. It is like a cloud that covers the soul, covers love, and compassion.*
*It makes it harder to see or feel one's true nature.*
*am the bridge between worlds.*
*I am the bridge between dimensions.*
*I have seen every single deed, every single error of humanity, and yet I still love them nevertheless.*
*My job, role, position—if you want to call it that—is to love them when they cannot love themselves, to give hope where hope has gone, to give embrace when another would not embrace, to give forgiveness when one could not even forgive themselves.*
*You see, I see all the grief, the anger, the malice, but I also see underneath it as well.*
*For every negative act, there is always a countermeasure, a wish, a desire, a true natural alliance to love and connection.*
*My role is to guide mankind. The universe only works via set rules.*
*It cannot apply a different outcome or even judgement to a situation.*
*It simply replays the energy that is being exerted.*
*I do not function in this way. I read between the lines and see what was really the underlying catalyst.*
*I am often thought of as a man. This is not 100% correct. I am the father of a man. I am a presence of energy. People who have seen me will view me through their own gauge. For them, it is easier to view me as a man.*
*For you it is a feeling, for you everything is a feeling, an energy source, a spirit if you like But yes you are correct, I am a masculine energy that contains the feminine*

*Today for you is a light one, it is a feeling to release, no more lessons to struggle through, no more feeling drained or unwell internally*
*This relationship, our relationship now is the most important one, due to the nature of my calling*
*For the world to see their doings, it must show on the face of man*
*For the world to heal, mankind must heal first.*
*I am here, to facilitate that process*
*For many, for those that can not do this for themselves*
*I am here*

## Chapter Summary

In this chapter, I shared my experiences with dark energy and entity interference and how these forces can impact a person's health and spiritual connection. I explained the different types of entities, including demonic and multi-dimensional beings, and how they attach to individuals. I discussed the challenges I faced in my own journey of dealing with entities and the importance of developing energetic boundaries and sovereignty. I also explored the connection between EBV and entity interference and how healing from the virus often requires addressing these darker forces. I shared cautionary tales about engaging with spiritual practices without proper understanding and protection and emphasised the importance of discernment and working with experienced healers in this realm.

## CHAPTER 7

# Transformation Is the Key to Healing EBV for Good

One of the greatest truths I learnt on my journey to healing myself, my family and hundreds of clients from EBV is that healing EBV goes hand in hand with transformation. In the early days of trying to improve my health and then heal from EBV, I didn't know this.

Like most people and the education available online and through books, I focused on healing my physical body through diet, Chinese herbs, supplements, etc. I had no idea that there were higher orders like my mind, brain structures, neurological stress, and spiritual connection that were all major contributors to my health decline and EBV.

So it's important to understand that healing Epstein-Barr virus is directly linked to your transformation. By now, you would have heard me speak or read about how EBV is an opportunistic virus that uses your stress responses against you. It's linked energetically to these triggers through the brain and through your past as well. EBV holds neurological structures in decline and affects stagnated consciousness levels. Often, people take a snapshot of their health, looking at it from this point in time and viewing EBV as just a virus, examining it physically but not linking it to why it was there in the first place.

When it comes to healing, you can't just get rid of something, like EBV, without understanding the real reason why it was there in the first place. You need to fix the holes, the places that allowed the disconnection, damage, and stress to occur. You fix those, and then you can heal. It's almost like we have to go back and heal those things in our past because there are lessons, and they are all interlinked. Epstein-Barr virus, energetically, holds so much information and association. So whatever that energetic association is for the person, you have to find those things and then heal them. It's like decoupling the stress that created it from the virus. Then, you can work with EBV and reduce it physically, but you have to release these triggers. Otherwise, people might find something that slightly reduces it in their body, but it just stays and waits until life happens again.

Often, people don't understand how changing their external life starts with changing internally because we create our reality. Up to this point, we've created it all.

It's almost like taking responsibility for why something is there. There's so much more to look at in life. Holding a higher elevated view gives you the path or potential to start making changes. For a person, EBV may symbolise not ever feeling loved. Maybe it symbolises a significant turning point in life where they were physically overrun. You have to find the reason why it could build up in the first place. Unfortunately, our lessons often come through pain and suffering.

Many people say illness is the best gift they ever received because it led them on a healing journey. We're all here to heal. That's the point.

So I want to explain something: the holographic brain and the holographic universe. The universe is actually holographic, and so is the brain. Scientifically, we know this because a number of studies conducted on rats' brains have proven it. In these studies, rats were taught to navigate a maze, after which parts of their brains were removed to observe the effects on neural networks and learned pathways. What was concluded was that no matter what part of the brain was cut out, the rat would still remember the maze.

Obviously, if too much was cut out, it was a different story. Although it proved that memory is holographic, that it crosses over the whole brain. The universe is also holographic, meaning a tiny piece of a hologram represents the whole picture. We represent the universe; we are a tiny piece but represent the whole. When we heal ourselves, we help to heal the collective, elevate consciousness, helping to heal the world and, ultimately, the universe. A world stuck in deep survival stress always thinks it doesn't have enough. When you heal, you show up differently. People start to serve at a higher level. When we raise our energetic vibration, things around us will shift; people will either fall away if they are not meant to be aligned, or they rise up to meet us. We are being asked to heal. This is what we are all here to do. At this point in the world, energetics are amplifying. This is why, if you're energetically attuned, both dark and light are getting more intense: The world needs to wake up and evolve. We are our own creators and destroyers. We need to look at our lives, but we need to look at the whole picture. It's not just this one snapshot of a virus causing health decline and disempowerment. There's a bigger story.

When I heal a person, the liver plays a huge role in reducing EBV. The liver is about transformation. I have to identify the key elements for transformation for that person. If EBV through the process hasn't reduced as much as I expected, it means there's a key piece missing for transformation in their life.

Change is the only constant thing, yet we get stuck. We always want to harmonise within ourselves and pull situations into us as a way to heal. It's about people tuning in to their highest form. Transformation is the key.

At one point, I was doing all the spiritual healing and transformation work. I realised that no matter what someone wanted to create in their life, I had to work on reducing EBV because it's symbolic of a lifetime of stress. It sits and waits. If you experience any stress or buildup, you start to derail. Our highest potential exists at the level of our soul. The truth of who we are and the reconnection to our divinity is the purpose of our existence.

EBV is about unlocking a person energetically, healing the life and history that have kept them stuck, and recycling fear and stress. We're here to heal ourselves. I've seen some people's trauma being solely linked to a bad legacy, their generational karma, what's been passed down. They chose to carry it forward, causing the biggest stress. It's about soul harmonisation, letting go of genetic integrity or potential. These things are stored at a cellular level in our body. Change your health, change your well-being. It's about setting ourselves free. It's about seeing restrictions as opportunities to grow and evolve. Sometimes, people come to me wanting a quick fix. Sorry, it doesn't work like that. The reconnection to self is the biggest gift of all.

I shared a lot about EBV being a multi-dimensional virus linked to high dark entities and how the virus is symbolic of the world we live in. This is why most people struggle with EBV, feeling helpless, confused, and overwhelmed. They are trying to deal with the physical symptoms of the virus, not the underlying reasons for its activity. EBV is symbolic of your life, energy, experiences, trauma, beliefs, genetics, DNA, generational lines, environment, and the collective of humanity. The medical industry doesn't have answers because they focus on symptoms, not the cause. The key to healing from EBV and other health issues is to live in alignment with your reason for being. True transformation can only be achieved by healing, aligning, and expanding your mind, body, energy, and soul. We all have a soul divine blueprint, an energetic template holding the truth of who we are at the soul level and how we are to express ourselves in the world. The world we live in has become polarised, dysfunctional, and disconnected from our highest truth. The disconnection from this template is a major catalyst for illness and disease.

Healing EBV is about more than physical transformation. Until more people work on their highest transformation, it will continue to get worse. The beautiful thing is everyone has a choice. Everyone can start a transformation journey. Everyone can start a healing journey.

By now, I hope you're starting to understand that EBV is linked to transformation. Even though I've created a process to heal people from EBV, all my clients have different life stories and reasons for why EBV increased and caused so much health decline. A person's stress has been the catalyst for EBV buildup. You have to look for the building blocks that create disconnection in the mind, body, and soul, as well as find the energetic representation of a client.

I could tell hundreds of stories of people I have worked with who have had unique stressful events in their lives that set the tone or anchor for their stress responses and life narratives. I'll see clients with C-PTSD from abusive relationships, those who were meant to love and support them the most. When let down in this way, it creates deep scars and unseen trauma. The brain's stress responses link love to being unsafe. Love becomes a stress. In a new healthy relationship, the brain links fear to it, creating disconnection and stress. This creates dysfunction over time.

This is why it's important to heal our past and unconscious programs, as they impact our mental, emotional, and physical health and how we respond to life. It's about changing that internal narrative and our life stories.

Healing these deep traumas and restrictions can even unlock our DNA. Our DNA is our blueprint for life, but trauma, limiting beliefs, and past conditioning can be stored at these deep levels in the body. This is the study of epigenetics and how these things can change and shape our gene expression, affecting how our body reads DNA sequences. The types of healing I speak about in this book restore energetic coding and unlock the potential within our cells and DNA.

When love and connection carry associated stress, it's conflicting because all we want is love and connection. You have to remove these deep underlying triggers, especially significant ones. Otherwise, a person's whole life becomes a stressor, and you cannot heal your body because it's linked to your DNA.

Why? Because EBV will recreate over and over when you are constantly stuck in this state of stress. I understand some people reading this book would have done a lot of work on themselves. Others might not have known that their unconscious brain programming and childhood events are directly linked to their stress responses and EBV buildup, creating so much decline years or decades later.

If you've done a lot of work, you'll have key information linked directly to EBV. I've seen people do endless healing work. I spoke more about this in the spiritual chapter.

But it's about finding the energetic associations to EBV directly. These will be key moments and key points in someone's life. When I speak to people looking to heal from EBV and other health issues, I ask them about their history. They'll often tell me about a time when their health really declined. You have to hear the undertone of the situation. You have to hear the energetic likeness or quality.

For example, I've been the healer to hundreds of successful business leaders in our program called The Evolved CEO. Due to their drive and determination to avoid mistakes and become successful, many run the perfectionist model program. They work hard to become successful, approaching every area of their business as problem solvers. This becomes their narrative for business and life. They strive for growth, momentum, and success in all areas, seeing stopping or resting as a failure.

This perfectionist model is universal, not just for business leaders. If I saw resting as a failure, I wouldn't want to do it. My brain would say rest creates worry and stress. Even if I rest and my external world looks peaceful and calm, internally, it's my internal gauge that sets the tone. Although your body may be resting, it's the mind that requires true rest.

As discussed in previous chapters, the mind controls the autonomic nervous system. An overactive mind constantly thinking and never truly resting is a huge problem. It means you wouldn't transition into your parasympathetic nervous system, even when you think you are resting or relaxing.

The deep unconscious program would be saying it's not safe to rest, that resting equals failure. You have to rewrite those programs in your life. The brain has to see relaxing as being safe and worry-free. Otherwise, this program can lead to severe illness and disease.

At another level, I see enormous neurological decline and mental health issues in highly driven, highly successful people, whether they are business leaders, entrepreneurs, or celebrities because they lose the ability to truly rest and repair themselves.

I also see people stepping away from high-stress environments, businesses, and even their life's work to put themselves first so they can heal and create more balance and a stress-free life. But the representation deep in their mind is failure, which simply engages more of a stress response.

I had another client who had a very stressful situation in their 20s. At the age of 20, we're really impressionable. We're still asking the world what it thinks of us. What we think somebody thinks of us is often not true.

This is where relationships or situations can be detrimental to someone's longevity or way of viewing themselves. My client had a job where the boss created so much stress, uncertainty, and unpredictability. This boss was on edge all the time, creating mental and emotional stress and uncertainty for employees. This was the time when they told me their health had declined significantly. They then told me more stories about when EBV reactivated—losing a job, financial struggles, stressful relationship dynamics, etc.

All of these events have an energetic representation linked back to that point in their life, which was the catalyst and main trigger for EBV. It represented "unpredictability." So running a program that meant unpredictable situations created instant stress, which meant that each time any event in life happened, it literally triggered the past response.

The way this client and many other people try to manage unpredictability or uncertainty is through control, leading the mind into a constant survival state, looking for any signs of threat or unpredictability.

Receiving an unexpected bill in the mail triggered an enormous mental and emotional stress response, pushing the body deeper into survival stress and allowing EBV to move through the body and reach the highest stages.

No matter what my client did to help herself heal from EBV, nothing was going to reduce it until the deepest underlying triggers were healed.

I worked with a beautiful lady in a loving relationship. They'd been together a long time, but there had been infidelity five to six years before we worked together. This created so much stress and disruption in their life. She was so hurt by the situation and really wanted to rebuild the foundations of her marriage, but she couldn't forgive or trust anymore. When she came to me, it was more for personal transformation and healing around these traumatic life events, but she had EBV at a very high level without knowing. The EBV represented that time in her life.

To create transformation, forgiveness, and give her trust and faith back, to embrace her marriage the way she wanted to, I had to heal EBV and reduce it from her body. At the same time, I worked on all of her stress responses from her past and what the marriage breakdown symbolised in her life. As long as EBV sat in her body, she could never forgive and rebuild her marriage because the virus held the resonance and memory associated with all her stress. She was constantly stuck in a stress state. As all these things healed—her beliefs, past hurts, and wounds—EBV reduced. Her mind and body healed, and she could elevate, expand, and forgive because they were all interlinked.

I've seen people receive kindness and love when they were unwell as a child, leading to an adult-based program where they constantly get sick, thinking they will only be loved when they are sick. Stories like this are more common than you'd imagine and extremely confusing when someone desperately wants to be healthy and happy, investing thousands of dollars trying to do so until they realise a powerful internal program is blocking their health and happiness.

When I heal people from Epstein-Barr virus, I have to hear their life stories. I have to understand why EBV built up in the first place. Some people ask if the virus is evil because I work with dark energy and dark entities. The answer is no.

EBV has morphed into something destructive, but it uses our own body and stress responses against us. Therefore, people have to be willing to look at their life, their past, and the role they played in it.

You have to be willing to look at the information or representations in your life around what you link stress and fear to.

I often say, "Stress is just a lazy word for fear."

We are becoming so busy, overrun, and living in a constant state of survival stress that fear or being in "fight or flight" has been normalised.

I used to constantly say, "I'm so stressed." But that statement told me nothing. It simply reinforced disempowerment and gave me no place to create change.

A better question was, "Why am I stressed?"

Looking at my life holistically, examining my mind and how I have created my own reality—these are the starting places for change. Becoming more aware of myself and accepting responsibility for everything in my life regardless of the situation—this is empowerment. So, I challenge you to look at the last time you had a flare-up. What was the tonality or energetic likeness of that situation? What did it represent? I guarantee if you find what that represents in your life, you can track it back to other points in time where that same quality appears, and there will be heightened stress responses around that.

Every time that quality shows up in your life, your brain does what it's designed to do. It literally goes looking for past history. It's like a computer. It goes back to see what it represents. Then, the mind decides how to respond to this situation. Even as an adult, I lived my life for a very long time, feeling like I was still a little girl. I felt like I had never really grown up. I was so fearful of many things.

One of the narratives or sayings I grew up with was, "Better the devil you know than the one you don't." I was scared of life. I looked confident and pushed myself, but it came from a stressed and scared place.

There's much more going on with Epstein-Barr virus and someone's health.

As the world heads deeper into health decline, illness, disease, and cancer, I find it interesting when people are diagnosed with a serious illness or cancer. It's almost like they are shocked they have it, almost as if it has simply just manifested in that moment in time. No one's health deteriorates that quickly. It has been years in the making, just like heightened levels of EBV. It's a body in continual decline, stuck in sympathetic nervous system dominance and unable to heal and repair itself.

The pathway to healing offers some of the most beautiful gifts you can ever receive.

When life is going well, unfortunately, people do not pay much attention to deeper issues. It's through suffering and struggle that we look and are given our lessons and an opportunity to address the underlying causes of decline. We are here to learn our lessons and evolve as a species.

Take the opportunity to look at your fear responses and identify the specific time and circumstances associated with the highest points of your health decline and links to EBV. What fears, beliefs, and programs are attached to these events? What is really holding you in a never-ending cycle of fear and ill health?

A mind filled with fear-based programs creates little space for higher wisdom. Epstein-Barr virus holds neurological pathways in decline, creating additional restriction and space for higher wisdom. This is the key to expanding your consciousness—not ramming more knowledge and information in your mind, but healing the mind and raising the energetic frequency to receive the wisdom of your higher self.

I once listened to a Buddhist monk speak. He had been a Buddhist monk for 25 years and lived a very peaceful and tranquil life. He then changed his life by moving back to Australia. He was still teaching but no longer living in a tranquil monastery. He also decided to foster a teenage boy, and as he told his story, he couldn't stop laughing. He said if he thought he had done all his work and resolved all his triggers, he was mistaken. It's easy to be at peace when our external world allows for peace and solitude, but the key to healing is finding the internal resolve to heal all our past wounds and triggers. Laughing, he said, "To be human means to be imperfect." He was now learning to do his journey differently, to use these experiences and the disharmony of bringing up a teenage boy as a way to continue growing and evolving.

I have teenage daughters, and I can tell you being a parent can be one of our biggest triggers. Our closest relationships, especially family and children, hold many of our learnings and lessons as they mirror our imperfections or push us to uncomfortable places. Often, I'll do healing work for people, and when I look at their relationships, it's never about the other person. It's always about what the other person represents.

I see people going to retreats, having all this beautiful, peaceful time to self-reflect. That's lovely, but the key to healing yourself is being able to do it in your day-to-day life.

I love this saying: "Peace does not mean being in a place where there is no noise, chaos, or hard work. It means being in the midst of all those things and still being calm in your heart."

My transformation is the thing I am most proud of in this lifetime—healing myself and reclaiming what was once lost. I'm not just talking about healing and well-being. Those things are important, but there are higher things to reclaim in the process. The mind, body, and soul are all interlinked. We are here to experience ourselves as whole.

Over time, I have learned so much about all these areas. It's fascinating how the human body and mind work, as well as the human spirit and our soul aspects. I have had to look deep within, challenge all my belief systems, and bring my spiritual gifts into physical manifestation.

I help people reorder their lives, heal old wounds, and release deep pain stored at all levels of their being.

I have healed so many layers in myself and my life. One of my biggest realisations was understanding my quality world pictures and representations in my life and what I equated success and failure to.

## Quality World Pictures

"Quality world pictures" refers to mental representations of what we equate success to in our lives. For me, it took a long time to work this out, and I needed to look at all areas of life.

We have relationships, which could be with a love partner, husband or wife, children, extended family, friends, and community. This represents love, connection, and belonging. Then we have health and well-being, including exercise, nutrition, and sleep, and what good health, happiness, and internal self-love look like for you.

We also have success, finances, lifestyle, impact, and legacy, which are very much external achievements or attainments that are important for our safety, security, and basic survival needs. So, we can have all these areas of life. And we have these things called quality world pictures around what success looks like for each of us in these areas. Now, what I find is that many people have outdated ideas, pictures, or views on their lives.

For example, with health and healing, maybe exercise. As people get older, their bodies change. As I write this book, I'm 45 years old. My body does not respond the way it used to. I can't push myself to the brink with exercise. I need to listen to my body. But people often have these ideas or pictures of what it looks like to succeed, and they are often outdated. They may exercise, eat, and drink the way they used to when they were younger, yet their bodies don't respond like they used to. It's almost like we have to update our quality world pictures and our views in all areas of our lives as we grow, evolve, and change. Otherwise, it sets a tone for failure. It's like running a race that can never be won.

Probably one of the most significant moments for me and my healing was when I realised I was playing an outdated world picture in a key area of my life over and over again. I've lived away from my family the whole time that I've had children. As you have read in my story, I had three kids under the age of five, which meant my life has been very stressful at times and quite lonely, too.

But again, these things were the building blocks for greatness and the foundation for me turning into the person I am now.

Back then, at this stressful point in my life, I had this story that I was always unsupported. And when I looked back on my idea of success as a mother, I realised I still held a picture from well before I had children or moved away from my hometown. This picture was of my family and my children having their grandparents in their lives day to day, plus me having the support of my family as I started my own. Due to my husband and I moving away from family in New Zealand to live in Australia before having children, it wasn't even an option or my reality.

Understanding that I was holding a quality world picture of family support being around me when I started my own family, but they weren't, was replaying a constant reminder in my mind that I was failing. That hugely significant area of my life constantly held stress for me because I realised my mind or my brain had these linked associations, and it wasn't even right. It was outdated, and yet it had an enormous effect on me, and I had no idea.

I see this often. I see this even in ideas for creating success. Maybe it's a business or career, and what does that look like? Because people have these outdated versions of themselves, when life changes, they change, yet many of these world pictures haven't been updated.

I've mentioned previously my fondness for the saying, "The unexamined life is not worth living." We often get in our own way so much with all these ideas or meanings and associations with different things in life. If we can become aware of some of these narratives, stories, or themes in our lives, it can be the starting place for viewing life differently and creating greater change and transformation.

## Chapter Summary

In this chapter, I've taken a deeper dive into the connection between healing from EBV and personal transformation. I've explained how EBV is linked to a person's life experiences, traumas, and belief systems and how addressing these underlying factors is key to lasting healing. Stories of clients who have undergone profound transformations by healing from EBV and the associated emotional and energetic blocks provided real-world examples of the ideas being presented. I discussed the importance of examining one's stress responses and outdated beliefs in creating genuine change. Healing is a personal journey of reconnecting with one's authentic self and soul purpose. The challenges we face along the way are opportunities for growth and evolution.

CHAPTER 8

# EBV Is a Collective Disease

EBV is a collective disease that is symbolic of the stress and dysfunction in humanity. You cannot heal from a collective disease virus while you operate, and you are constantly energetically pulled into the low vibration of the collective. This is why healing from EBV and preventing its return is about transformation, healing, and alignment in your mind, body, and soul.

95% of the world's population is stuck in deep survival stress, but we have normalised this because the collective is in it. In this state, we feel like we don't have enough, constantly recycling the past, and stuck in the duality of the physical world.

The world lives within a delicate balance of many microorganisms, from our external world to our internal world. Once upon a time, EBV was in balance within our bodies and didn't attack our minds and bodies' glands, organs, systems and structures like it does now. But due to the amount of stress, toxicity, dysfunction and decline within the world, over time, EBV has adapted and morphed into a multi-dimension virus that causes so much destruction. As you have learnt by now, it uses our bodies and our internal stress responses against us, feeding off increased levels of toxicity and stress. This is why new viruses like COVID-19 heightened EBV, as they both target the weakest point in the existing dysfunction in each individual's mind and body.

EBV represents more than a virus. It's symbolic of a world on the brink of unprecedented stress disorder and disconnection. It's also symbolic of a lifetime of stress, generational stress disorder, and disconnection passed down through DNA.

The rate at which EBV chews up valuable resources within our bodies is unprecedented. This symbolises humanity and how we are doing this very thing to Mother Earth by depleting her natural resources and with pollution and destruction.

We are here to heal. We are here to evolve. We are here to resolve our karmas, our lessons, and all the things that come mainly in the shape of trauma, disconnection, and suffering. When we do not address these areas within ourselves, they create more disharmony in our mind, body, and soul, which fuels an unruly virus like EBV to thrive and create more dysfunction and disconnection, resulting in more health issues and concerns. Often, people's health journeys lead to newfound awakenings. The world is being asked to heal. Humans are being forced to evolve, but as a collective, we are not. Mental and emotional health is on the rise across all age groups, and collective diseases like EBV will continue to thrive in the disharmony and dysfunction we have all created.

We are all responsible for the world you see today, and it's not all bad. People are doing more amazing things for the world and humanity than ever before, but it's not enough because the majority of the World, the collective, is either in survive or decline—not expansion and evolving.

As discussed in previous chapters, we are spiritual beings having a human experience, and every individual being is not here by mistake; we have a one-in-a-billion chance of being conceived, and part of this journey is our soul and our soul's purpose. This comes with choice and free will.

The physical will mirror the spiritual. There is always an interplay between dimensions and orders. It has used our bodies against us. EBV is like a parasite that needs a host to duplicate itself. And again, it's symbolic of humans on Earth. When a person is stuck in deep survival stress, they feel like they don't have enough. We are living in a world of instant gratification, constantly seeking external resources to fill a widening gap within.

This overarching need for more is directly linked to how we are chewing up resources at an unprecedented rate. It's exactly the same as what EBV does in the body. And then we look to fill this void through the external world, but the truth is it's an internal disconnection that also allows EBV to chew up all the resources in your body, which results in a compounding effect of more internal disconnection and health decline.

The more we are disconnected internally, the more we feel disconnected in our daily lives, and the more we disconnect from our spiritual aspects and the truth of who we are, the more EBV will use your body against us.

As I have discussed throughout this book, there are hundreds of symptoms of illness and disease that affect an enormous percentage of the world's population, including cancers, organ dysfunction, sympathetic nervous system dominance, stress, fatigue, and poor sleep. The list goes on and on. Yet, they are all symptoms of years of decline, much like the dysfunction we see in the world—so many symptoms of years of decline and ignorance. Imbalance and dysfunction are the compounding effects of the world we live in, and EBV is associated at the deepest level with 95% of all health issues I've ever seen.

Our past traumas, emotions, genetic karmas, genetic potential, and environmental changes shape our gene expression. We are designed to do this. This is called Epigenetics. All living organisms on Earth recreate themselves over and over.

They change to match their environment. This is evolution and exactly what Epstein-Barr virus has done. It's pre-programmed to reactivate, build up, and recreate itself over and over. So when I heal EBV, I have to heal all the reasons why it built up in the first place and then energetically recode the virus back to its original state before it morphed out of control. This stops the reactivation process from building back up again unless a person seriously and intentionally de-evolves themselves.

When I started working with EBV, I had foundational knowledge from my advanced platform of Advanced Holistic Kinesiology. It gave me the foundation to work in-depth with human anatomy, organs, glands, neurological structures, and functions. It was only through working in people's energetics that I was able to track the stages, percentages, and severity of Epstein-Barr virus, giving me a clear picture and knowledge of how it affects the body so severely, including the pathways it takes and the destruction in the body. This allowed me to reverse engineer and create a healing process and protocol that takes it from the highest stage all the way back to the starting place of each organ and gland to deep neurological decline and compromise.

This allowed me to formulate an in-depth healing process to help a person reduce and heal from EBV at the deepest of levels.

Although I was reducing it in people's bodies, I knew that even if I reduced it, at some point, it would build back up. There was a process to reduce it, not just physically but energetically. There are stored associations, stored energetic memories, specific stress-related responses, trauma, and very specific times in a person's life that have all equated to this imbalance. All of this needed to be addressed at the same time. Even then, it was only a matter of time before it could rebuild itself with any stressful life event. And let's be honest, life happens. It is full of uncertainty, ups and downs. It's simply the way it works.

Then, one day, I had an epiphany. I realised that if I reduced it enough, and if something used to be in balance, it could always be brought back into balance again. I was working with frequency at the time, very high multi-dimensional frequencies with heightened healing abilities. As I had this realisation, it led to me being shown and guided to higher vibration frequencies capable of returning order to a structure, to a living organism, to a virus. I created a new energetic process that recoded the energetics of Epstein-Barr virus.

As EBV holds an energetic program, it feeds off stress and recreates itself over and over. It's the same as our own minds and bodies. We can end up running programs that do not serve us. We get stuck in preprogrammed ways of being. We almost get stuck in a stress loop, and our body just gets used to living in that state. EBV carries these energetics, too, because it's morphed and changed, and it's ended up being programmed to create more and more dysfunction.

There are so many interlinks because everything is interconnected. This is why when we change our internal landscape from stress to balance, from trauma to healing. That is why, for a person to be in optimal health and well-being, they have to find the true underlying cause and heal from that. In 95% of cases, EBV is the deepest underlying cause, but again, it's not one-dimensional. To heal from EBV, you have to hear and know all the pieces of information to dismantle it correctly for you as an individual. This is where the elements of healing, to live in alignment with our spiritual connection, are so important. And it's almost impossible to do this if you are controlled and deeply connected to the collective.

If I'm only looking at one piece of the puzzle or one dimension of a person, it would never make sense, and this is why I see thousands of people with EBV blood tests and still no solution or answers to how to get rid of it for good.

EBV is symbolic of an individual being so oriented by the physical world. It's like we haven't even realised how much of our internal world has been suffering. EBV is symbolic of a world in dysfunction and imbalance, along with humanity's interplay with Mother Earth and the physical being as a mirror for the spiritual. There's always an interplay. The world is shifting, changing, evolving, and we're being asked to shift with her.

If you think the divide between people being unwell versus being healthy is large now, it's just going to get bigger and bigger as people are de-evolving at a rapid rate, and only a small percentage are truly waking up, doing the correct healing work for themselves to then help shift the collective vibrational energy.

It's hard to even tell now who is unwell and who is not. People don't really wear it on their face like they used to; it's internal. This is why it's hard to judge other people's lives. We look at all these other people, and we see their external representation, but it's not a true gauge of what's actually going on. I can tell you now that I have done energetic audits for people who are extremely sick internally and energetically, yet they look sensational externally in their appearance. It used to shock me when I would get a Zoom energy audit call booking and an assessment of a person's health issues, only to have them show up to my Zoom call looking so beautiful and healthy. This doesn't shock me anymore, as the saying "you can't judge a book by its cover" is never more true than when understanding where a person's health is at.

I've heard a lot of talk about the world shifting to 5D. She has always been in 5D. It is us that need to shift, and reality is splitting. It's the story of the healed and the unhealed. People are stuck by the limitations of their own minds, the reality that they were born into, and the reality that they choose to keep. I see people looking to external things to offer rebalancing. They may purchase products like necklaces for sacred geometry to protect their energetic field; however, it's not as simple as just wearing a necklace. This may offer support, yet we have sacred geometry within our energetic matrices. We actually need to realign at these higher energetic levels to be in optimal health.

It is true that everything has to be created in the spiritual before it will manifest into the physical. However, I see a lot of spiritual healers and truth seekers amplifying more and more disconnection in the world.

You see, there is so much conflict and duality at the moment. People will think that they are on the right side of something, for or against it. It does not matter what side you are on. It is all the same: the flip side of a coin. Duality only exists at the fourth dimension, the level of our minds.

I don't function from the collective. The collective will make you sick. There were times when I opened up to more people through doing EBV, and it actually made me quite unwell because I was focusing on who I couldn't help. It made me feel really sad. I had to do a lot of work on myself, and I realised I had dropped my energetics down to the collective level. I see people stuck in stories about past events and situations that may have negatively affected them in the physical world. They're still living their life from past events, even calling themselves truth seekers. Trying to "right" a perceived "wrong," stuck in information overload or conspiracy theories. Those pathways keep people stuck, linked deeply in low vibrational collective energy yet constantly justifying they are on the side of the truth. There are no sides—dark and light co-exist—this is the illusion of the mind, the ego, and keeps people trapped in duality and needing validation from the collective. The majority of the collective wouldn't have a clue what true world agendas or orders look like.

I do a lot of work at high multi-dimensional levels related to Earth grid interference, humanity's evolution, and levels like the Galactic Federation of Light. This is all due to my specialised gifts with entities. There are things I'm not allowed to speak about. But I would never play guessing games. A lot of people in the world are doing this. People have naive views of light and dark and think it is as simple as light opposing dark.

Light and dark actually work together, depending on the agenda. It is not as black and white as people think. Going down these pathways and rabbit holes simply creates more distractions and restrictions for people as they get drawn in and get stuck at the level of the collective mind.

We are here to heal ourselves. We are here to experience ourselves as separate. We are here to elevate, to live our divinity, and to rise above it. That's how we actually help to heal the world. I helped many people through COVID-19, such as helping business leaders elevate themselves. It didn't matter what was going on in the world. You live in alignment; you step out of deep survival stress, you heal yourself, you show up differently, and you start to serve at a higher level.

I love to work with people who are serious about healing and expansion. They want to heal themselves so they can show up differently in the world and make a bigger impact—to serve at a higher level. Create things that the world actually needs rather than just chewing up more resources because we think that we don't have enough.

Those are the real stories about healing. Knowing we're all energetically different. Where does your power lie? Some people, again, talk about all living in our heart space. No. For some people, it's from their solar plexus' "personal power" or from their wisdom. Again, trying to match up with whatever the collective is saying or doing. It may not be exactly right for you. It's about living in alignment with your divinity. It's about manifesting and creating from that place. When we live in alignment with that, we are in alignment with human expansion. When we are in alignment with human expansion, we will be in alignment with the Earth. When the Earth shifts, we will shift with her. We will be on our correct path of progression. And when we're living from that place of divinity, the sixth dimension is living your divinity and integrating it into your life. And when you honour that, that is abundance, that is health, that is all these things, and they come from this internal connection point.

The collective needs to heal, and in order for the collective to heal, the individual needs to first heal themselves.

Epstein-Barr virus has many collective interplays. Our engagement and interplay with the second dimension (2D) is one of the biggest threats to our existence as a collective. As mentioned in Chapter 5, the second dimension (2D) is known as the Telluric realm. It is an unseen world, one of microorganisms, parasites and viruses, but it is also one of minerals, crystals, and the intricate life forms and elements that make up the ecosystems of Mother Earth. We are being heavy-handed, taking more resources than we need to fuel many frivolous needs, wants, and desires without thought of the consequences, creating imbalance and instability in these delicate realms.

Epstein-Barr virus is part of this unseen and very powerful world, one that we often take for granted. These unseen worlds, when taken out of balance, can create many imbalances and restrictions across all areas of life, across all areas of a person's being. Did you know we live on a planet of viruses? We update through the virome. We are actually only 10% human, with one human cell for every ten impostor cells. Even within our own bodies, there is a delicate ecosystem of organisms coexisting. I often have people ask me if Epstein-Barr virus is a dark entity. No, it is a virus that has recreated itself because the landscape where it resided changed. This is evolution, organisms changing and adapting over time to their environment.

The real question we should be asking ourselves is how to change our internal landscape back to one of harmony and balance. Many of the answers are provided in the previous chapters. Many of the dimensions will cross-reference one another: Just as everything in the ecosystem is interlinked, so are the dimensions, parasites, and microorganisms. Even viruses that hold destructive abilities go hand in hand with dark entities and dark energy engagement. As a world, we need to stop looking at everything in isolation, only seeing one issue at a time. Many issues breed from the same foundation.

In time, I have no doubt that there will be many other viruses that change their orientation and take advantage of a dysfunctional and stressed environment, the environments that we create. In time, there will be many more dark faces among the unseen worlds. The key is to unify worlds, orders, and dimensions and restore balance. This is what creates stability.

To create more internal balance, many keys lie at a collective level. We should be asking many questions not just of ourselves, but also seeking to maintain a more balanced environment.

The real question we should be asking ourselves is how to change our internal landscape and how to recreate a more balanced environment internally. The world should be asking the same. As all life needs to be restored to hold more balance and harmony, our world is forever changing. There will be more and more viruses over time that change to meet the ever-shifting environments inside and out. Epstein-Barr virus is symbolic of many things, including our pathways to decline.

## Chapter Summary

In this final chapter, I have explored the collective aspects of EBV and how it reflects the broader imbalances and dysfunctions in our world. I explained how EBV is symbolic of humanity's disconnection from nature, spirit, and our true selves and how healing from the virus requires a shift in consciousness both individually and collectively. I discussed the role of the second dimension (the Telluric realm) in the ecosystem of life and how our actions impact these unseen worlds. I emphasise the importance of asking questions, both of ourselves and of the world around us, in order to restore balance and harmony. In conclusion, I have encouraged readers to take responsibility for their own healing journey and to recognise the power they have to create change, not just in their own lives but in the world as a whole.

**Channelled Message** (divine guidance that speaks poetically, awakening a deep, heightened sense of knowing and truth within.)

*The earth's frequencies are shifting*
*We are being called forth to elevate*
*To rise above the collective for this is the only place of true and lasting alignments*
*Light and dark competing for the same space, constraints of the mind, constraints of the collective mind oppose many things*
*Resource depletion in the form of micro landscapes in ability to renew themselves*
*The external mirrors the internal*
*The physical mirrors the spiritual*
*Just as depletion can occur on more levels than conscious awareness would have you belief*
*The world is speeding up, new frequencies added to an already faltering frequency*
*Knowledge growing and with it creating less and less space for the eternal most powerful knowledge base of all*
*Universal reordering*
*Generational karma playing through one lineage, a world in decline, a world that each new generation has to re navigate.*

# Conclusion

Wow, what a journey it has been, learning, healing, recoding, and understanding the deepest truths behind Epstein-Barr virus.

In the world of medical research, EBV remains a mystery. It has so many links and interplays with various illnesses and diseases. This is why researching only one or two dimensions of a human being means you'll never get the full picture and the truth behind a virus as destructive as EBV. I feel incredibly blessed that my extremely hard journey to healing and spiritual awakening led me to master the truth behind EBV and create healing processes that not only heal a person from EBV but also stop the reactivation process, giving people the platform to heal other illnesses and health concerns.

I hope that after reading this book, you have gained much more clarity on EBV as a multi-dimensional virus that needs to be healed and harmonised on all levels of your being.

Knowing there is an order to healing EBV and understanding that every single person's story and reason behind EBV building up in them is unique, it is important to find the cause behind why EBV built up in the first place.

I encourage you to think back to key events in your past where you believe your health declined. It could have been a traumatic event in childhood or a major stress event personally or professionally.

Identifying these key events will help to create a pathway to create more healing and change. It could be a turning point to unlocking important information linked to Epstein-Barr virus activation and to help unwind the virus.

I want to thank you and congratulate you on reading my book. Some people tell me it contains the most profound information they have ever read about EBV, while others may find it hard to process as it may challenge some of their deepest belief systems. Either way, I hope this book has provided you with more insights and strategies to advance your own healing and transformation journey.

You are here for a reason. I know the journey, at times, can feel insurmountable. I have been there struggling for survival, struggling to reclaim my divine rights, sovereign presence, and always searching to come home to myself.

Healing can almost become a job in itself, but believe me, there are key moments in time. Key information, when found and realigned, creates a cascading effect through out mind, body and soul. It's your soul's purpose to evolve as an individual. This means doing the work to heal, to align, and expand into the highest version of yourself. Although my journey has been unbearable at times, and I wanted to stop, quit, and shut myself down, this was just not possible. In the book, I mentioned a saying that helped me through the hardest times, the most intense dark nights of the soul: "When you're going through hell, don't stop."

You have unique gifts; everyone has unique gifts. It is your soul's pathway to unlock those gifts so you can be part of an evolving society and the collective. Remember, healing from EBV goes hand in hand with transformation, and transformation is about unlocking the reason why you are here.

I want to encourage you to be highly motivated in your journey of healing and transformation. Change is challenging, and the greater the change, the greater the challenge. But I promise you, whenever there is darkness, there is a new level of light waiting on the other side. If you are determined to heal and evolve, you will find the answers.

# A Special Thank You

As a special thank you for buying my book, I'm excited to offer you additional resources!

If you want to take the next step in your journey to healing EBV and transforming your life, I invite you to access my FREE Community, where you will access my Truth about EBV Mini-course, healing resources, tools and more.

I wish you all the best in your healing journey
Much Love
Tracey

# THANK YOU FOR READING MY BOOK!

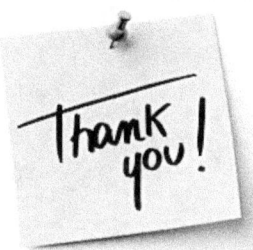

## ACCESS MY FREE COMMUNITY &
## THE TRUTH ABOUT EBV MINI-COURSE

To help you gain more knowledge on *The Truth Behind Epstein-Barr Virus* plus access to additional learnings, resources, and a community to support your healing and transformation journey! Please scan the QR code for the above gifts!

**Scan the QR Code:**

*I appreciate your interest in my book and value your feedback as it helps me improve future versions of this book. I would appreciate it if you could leave your invaluable review on Amazon.com with your feedback. Thank you!*

www.ingramcontent.com/pod-product-compliance
Lightning Source LLC
Chambersburg PA
CBHW070329010526
44107CB00004B/463